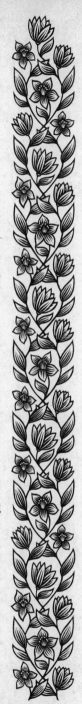
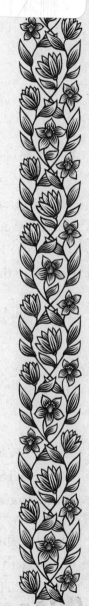

Llewell

Herbal Almanac
2009

© 2008 Llewellyn Worldwide
Llewellyn is a registered trademark
of Llewellyn Worldwide.
Editing/Design: Ed Day
Interior Art: © Fiona King,
excluding illustrations on pages 2–4,
which are © Mary Azarian
Cover Photos: © Digital Vision, © Brand X,
© Digital Stock, © Photodisc
Cover Design: Kevin R. Brown

You can order annuals and books
from *New Worlds*, Llewellyn's
catalog. To request a free copy
call toll-free: 1-877-NEW WRLD, or visit our
website at http://subscriptions.llewellyn.com.

ISBN 978-0-7387-0723-5
Llewellyn Worldwide
2143 Wooddale Drive
Woodbury, MN 55125-2989

CLINTON PUBLIC LIBRARY
CLINTON, IOWA
52732

253 9796

596 M

262 1976355

BAT

8/8/08

7.00

DISCARD

Table of Contents

Growing and Gathering Herbs

Culinary Herbs

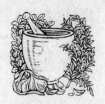

Herbs for Health

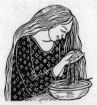

Herbs for Beauty

CLINTON PUBLIC LIBRARY
CLINTON, IOWA
52732

Herb Crafts

Herb History, Myth, and Lore

Introduction to Llewellyn's
Herbal Almanac

The herbal landscape is an ever-evolving one. The slow warming of our planet has temperate climates creeping toward the poles, while consumer trends prompt more immediate changes. But through it all, home-grown herbs still make a lasting impact. Llewellyn's *2009 Herbal Almanac* takes a look at the year-round effects of herbs, re-examining the research on uses of herbs as medicine, as culinary spices, as cosmetics, and more. This year we once again tap into practical, historical, and just plain enjoyable aspects of herbal knowledge—using herbs to enhance the health of infants and adults; discovering new ways to streamline your gardening tasks; developing home-based hobbies; and, of course, trying out new recipes for old standbys such as pestos, enticingly aromatic breads, and classic seasoning combinations that enhance your personal favorites. And we bring to these pages some of the most innovative and original thinkers and writers on herbs.

Growing, preparing, and using herbs allows us to focus on the old ways—when men and women around the world knew and understood the power of herbs. Taking a step back to a simpler time is important today as the pace of everyday life quickens and demands more and more of our energy—leaving precious little room for beauty, good food, health, love, and friendship. This state of affairs is perhaps not terribly surprising considering so many of us are out of touch with the beauty, spirituality, and health-giving properties of the natural world. Many of us spend too much of our lives rushing about in a technological bubble. We forget to focus on the parts of life that can bring us back into balance and harmony.

Though it's getting more difficult, you can still find ways to escape the rat race once in a while. People are still striving to make us all more aware of the uplifting, beautiful ways that herbs can affect our lives. In the 2009 edition of the *Herbal Almanac*, the various authors pay tribute to the ideals of beauty and balance in relation to the health-giving and beautifying properties of herbs. Whether it comes in the form of a new and natural hair-care regimen, a way to improve digestion, simple tips for healthy travel, or a new favorite recipe, herbs can clearly make a positive impact in your life.

Herbs are the perfect complement to the power of the mind, an ancient tool whose time has come back around to help us restore balance in our lives. More and more people are using them, growing and gathering them, and studying them for their enlivening and healing properties. We, the editors and authors of this volume, encourage the treatment of the whole organism—of the person and of the planet—with herbal goodness.

Note: The old-fashioned remedies in this book are historical references used for teaching purposes only. The recipes are not for commercial use or profit. The contents are not meant to diagnose, treat, prescribe, or substitute consultation with a licensed health-care professional. Herbs, whether used internally or externally, should be introduced in small amounts to allow the body to adjust and to detect possible allergies. Please consult a standard reference source or an expert herbalist to learn more about the possible effects of certain herbs. You must take care not to replace regular medical treatment with the use of herbs. Herbal treatment is intended primarily to complement modern health care. Always seek professional help if you suffer from illness. Also, take care to read all warning labels before taking any herbs or starting on an extended herbal regimen. Always consult medical and herbal professionals before beginning any sort of medical treatment—this is particularly true for pregnant women.

Herbs are powerful things; be sure you are using that power to achieve balance. Llewellyn Worldwide does not participate in, endorse, or have any authority or responsibility concerning private business transactions between its authors and the public.

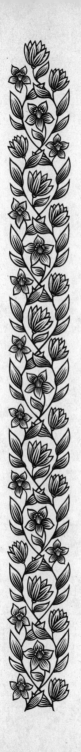

Growing
and
Gathering
Herbs

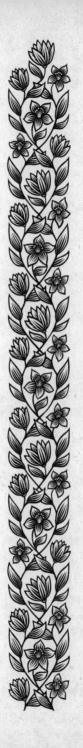

Lazy Gardens
for Busy Bodies

❧ by Elizabeth Barrette ❧

Everybody loves a garden and
fresh garden herbs. But everybody hates weeding—and not
everybody has good soil for a garden,
or the ability to dig it. Fortunately,
there are some alternatives. All the garden types described here are great for
gardeners whose soil is very poor, thin,
rocky, or otherwise less than ideal for
growing herbs. These gardens are also
very easy to establish, making them a
perfect choice for busy gardeners who
aren't up to heavy garden labor.

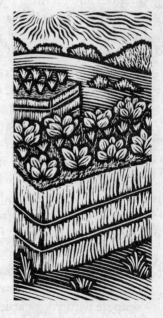

All of these "lazy gardens" have
one thing in common: they are built
up from the soil surface, rather than
dug down into it. Each uses a different method to create and contain a
good growing medium for your various herbs, flowers, and vegetables.
They also come in different sizes for
gardeners with various amounts of
space. Let's explore the options.

The Lasagna Garden

The lasagna garden uses multiple layers of organic material to create a bed for growing plants. Unlike traditional raised beds, however, the lasagna garden does not require a truckload of expensive topsoil or the tedious removal of existing sod. Instead it uses a solid base layer to smother grass and weeds. Then, it stacks up successive layers of different organics, which will eventually decompose into fine soil. You can build your lasagna garden with or without a defined border. One terrific advantage to this method is that you can get most or all materials for a lasagna garden free!

This type of garden is good for leafy herbs like sorrel, thyme, or lettuce. Plants with a shallow- to moderate-root system, such as asparagus and garlic, do especially well in a lasagna garden, too. After a year or two, the layers will break down into loose, rich compost. Add more organic matter to the top and keep going—but now you can plant crops with deeper roots such as potatoes and carrots.

You can assemble a lasagna garden either in the spring or in the fall. If you make yours in the spring, you can plant in it immediately. This works best if you include plenty of compost or topsoil in your layers and avoid using anything that might contain live weed seeds. If you make your garden in the fall, you can cover it with black plastic and allow it to "cook" until spring. This will kill any undesirable seeds and break down much of the organic matter into rich compost. However, southern gardeners may plant immediately in a fall garden to take advantage of the cool phase of their growing season.

Your lasagna garden is only as good as what you put into it. Never use organic matter that has been treated with artificial herbicides, pesticides, fertilizers, or other chemicals. Those things aren't good for your plants, or you, or the Earth. Anything that may contain live weed seeds, such as uncomposted barn litter, should go in the lower layers so the weeds won't survive to compete with your garden plants.

Many different types of organic matter are suitable for a lasagna garden, including but not limited to:

- Paper bags, cardboard, or newspaper (no glossy or colored paper)
- Coir or peat moss
- Corn stalks, chopped corncobs, bark chips, twigs, or small branches
- Chopped leaves, grass clippings, straw, hay, seaweed, or sawdust
- Barn litter, animal manure, bone meal, or wood ash
- Compost or topsoil

Notice the grouping. The first set of choices would go on the bottom of your garden to smother grass and weeds. The middle layers would consist of choices from the middle of the list, varying density and richness. The top layer provides a good starter medium for your garden plants or seeds. Finally, adding a layer of relatively inert mulch—such as straw or bark chips—between your plants will retain moisture and discourage weeds.

To Start a Lasagna Garden, Follow These Steps:

1. Study your yard to find a place that gets the right amount of sun. Most herbs need at least six hours of direct sun per day.

2. Mow or trample any existing grass or weeds.

3. Use a rope or hose to outline the shape of your garden.

4. Set out a wide pan of water and a stack of newspapers (or other base material). Wet the newspaper a few sheets at a time and spread them over the base of your garden outline. Cover the whole space with several layers of newspaper, overlapping sheet edges by at least two inches.

5. Spread two inches of absorbent material (coir or peat moss) over the newspaper to retain moisture and beneficial bacteria.

6. Spread about four inches of low-density material, such as corn stalks or twigs. This aids drainage and aeration.

7. Add two- to four-inch layers of other organic materials such as chopped leaves, grass clippings, barn litter, and compost.

8. For best results, alternate high-carbon layers (chopped leaves, straw) with high-nitrogen layers (fresh grass, animal manure) . Including some layers of compost or topsoil will add beneficial organisms. Also, moisten any dry matter after you spread it. The garden should be damp, but not soggy.

9. Top with four inches (or a bit more) of compost or rich topsoil to plant in. The total stack of layers should be about eighteen to twenty-four inches thick.

10. You can plant immediately, and cover any gaps between plants with mulch; or, cover with black plastic to let the garden decompose before planting.

Hay, It's a Garden!

This is exactly what it sounds like: you take a bale of straw or hay and plant things in it. The best is wheat straw, which contains the fewest unwelcome seeds. You'll want bales bound with synthetic twine, if possible; wire rusts through and can snag skin, while natural twine rots quickly. Bales last at least one full growing season, sometimes two. After that—just break them up and fork the remains onto your compost heap!

Bale gardens are good for deep-rooted leafy herbs like sage. They're also ideal for basil, cilantro, chervil, and parsley; some people use them for growing lettuce, mesclun, or other salad mixes. Nasturtiums and other edible flowers add color. Bales make a spectacular display when planted with weeping, creeping, or running herbs such as strawberry, creeping thyme, or prostrate rosemary. (Some of those can be planted in holes all over the sides of the bale as well as the top.) They provide a way to contain enthusiastic runners like mint, too. For vegetables, consider peppers, tomato, bush bean, cucumber, and watermelon. Avoid planting any tall crops (like corn) or root crops (like parsnip) in bales.

You can make a bale garden as small as one bale, or as large as you want. Think of the bales like blocks or legos, and you can see the possibilities for building low walls, mazes or labyrinths, simple symbols, or just a garden patch of perfect rows. They are especially convenient for people who can't bend over easily. But put them where you want them to stay, because once they get wet, they're too heavy and fragile to move.

To Start a Bale Garden, Follow These Steps:

1. Buy some bales, preferably wheat straw. You can usually get them from a local farmer, farmer's market, or farm supply store; or check your newspaper for classified ads.

2. Choose a location that gets enough sun for your herbs, preferably six or more hours per day. Position your bales with the bindings horizontal and the straws vertical for best root penetration. Don't cut the binding, or the bales will fall apart; using a stake at each end helps the bales keep their shape.

3. Soak the bales thoroughly using a garden hose. Continue to water once or twice daily to keep them moist for one to two weeks. This allows them to start decomposing into a suitable growth medium. They'll heat up during that process, so you don't want to plant anything yet—but it will help kill the wheat seeds. Some wheat may sprout anyway; you can weed it out if you want.

4. Pour on some natural, liquid fertilizer such as fish emulsion, liquid seaweed, compost tea, or worm tea.

5. Scratch over the top surface of the straw with a three-tined hand fork. Add at least half a dozen earthworms per bale. You can dig them from your yard, or just buy some at a bait shop.

6. Place two to four inches of planting medium on top of each bale. (You'll need less for starting seeds than for transplanting seedlings.) Use compost, potting soil, topsoil, or a half-and-half blend of topsoil and either compost or rotted manure. Mist the planting medium to moisten.

7. Sow seeds directly in the top layer of planting medium. To transplant seedlings, first thrust a trowel through the planting medium and into the bale itself. Pull back sharply to create a

hole. (If necessary you can wiggle the trowel or scoop out some of the rotting straw to enlarge the hole.) Push the seedling gently into the hole, slip the trowel out, and firm the medium around the stem.

8. Once bales get wet, they never really dry out. However, you'll need to water your garden until the plants are well established. After that, water occasionally if the weather is really hot and dry or if the plants start to wilt. Fertilize as needed with natural, liquid fertilizer.

The Lazy Tater Garden

Here is an easy way to grow herbs without straining your back: put them in pots. For this, you need a collection of medium to large containers and some suitable growth medium. This is an ideal choice for root crops (ginger, horseradish, potatoes, etc.) and herbs that spread aggressively (mint, strawberries, etc.). It also works when you have plants with many different soil and water requirements, but minimal space to grow them. Each pot can have a different growth medium if necessary.

What makes this type of garden easy is the use of containers. They require a little extra attention for watering if you don't set up an automatic system; but they require little weeding. To harvest the root crops at the end of the season, you simply dump out the pots! The potting medium will fall away, leaving the roots for you to pick up and dust off. Leafy crops like mint can be picked as desired in the ordinary way.

Here's How You Set Up This Kind of Garden:

1. Decide what you want to grow; this will determine what type of growth medium you need. You can buy a commercial potting mix or make your own from such ingredients as sand, peat moss, topsoil, vermiculite, compost, rotted manure, and so forth.

2. Obtain some containers. They should be at least one gallon in size, on up to however large you can comfortably handle. Ten gallons is a good maximum if you aren't sure—full pots get pretty

heavy. Matching containers are better than mixed ones, and they don't need to be fancy. Sometimes you can get empty plastic pots from a nursery in late spring or early summer free of charge.

3. Arrange the containers in a configuration that will be easy for you to tend. A three-by-three square works for most people. Rows two or three pots wide can be as long as you wish, and can form interesting shapes, such as a star or labyrinth.

4. Fill all the containers with potting medium. If the medium is dry, moisten it carefully. It should be about the consistency of a damp sponge.

5. Buy your plants and seeds. Read labels carefully—sometimes you can find recommendations for which varieties grow well in containers.

6. Plant your garden. Seeds should be pressed gently into the surface of the growth medium. You can sow radishes, carrots, and other small-seeded root crops rather densely, and thin them out later. (This discourages weeds and allows you to select the healthiest plants to keep.) Sow root crops such as garlic, ginger, onion, horseradish, or potato more sparingly. One root section per pot is enough, unless you're using very large pots. Most runners, like mint, should be planted one to a pot. Strawberries, however, don't mind crowding and can be planted more densely; check the label for recommended spacing guidelines for the variety you've bought. Water gently after planting.

7. If you are using very large containers, such as half-barrels or pots intended for miniature trees, then you should top the growth medium with a layer of mulch. (Keep the mulch a couple of inches away from your seedlings or seeds.) It will reduce the need for weeding and watering.

8. For maintenance, water frequently but make sure the root crops don't get waterlogged. If your growth medium contains manure or compost, your garden may not need supplemental feeding. Otherwise, it probably will. Natural liquid fertilizer is a better choice than synthetic, and easy to apply. Fish emulsion, liquid seaweed, worm tea, or compost tea all work very well.

9. Harvest your garden by dumping out the pots. Pick up the roots. Shovel the leftover growth medium onto your compost heap if you have one; if you don't, give it to a friend who does. Containers can be reused if you wash them in a soap or bleach solution (to kill plant diseases and pests) then stack them away for next spring.

No matter how you get started, all gardens are a special labor of love. Herbs, vegetables, and flowers spring from the dark soil to bring us bright flowers and delicious flavors. Invite some friends over to help construct your garden—show them some ideas from this article—and you can add some personal touches and a community spirit by working together. It's a lot more fun when you can commiserate as you shovel manure into the lasagna garden. Dragging around hay bales is less work when you've got five or six people to share the work, and that way you can try different patterns until you find one that you all like. With containers, everyone can have one to paint and plant. It's a lovely way to spend an afternoon!

For Further Reading

Lanza, Patricia. *Lasagna Gardening: A New Layering System for Bountiful Gardens: No Digging, No Tilling, No Weeding, No Kidding!* Rodale Books, 1998. A simple, thorough, step-by-step introduction to layered gardening techniques.

Lanza, Patricia. *Lasagna Gardening with Herbs: Enjoy Fresh Flavor, Fragrance, and Beauty with No Digging, No Tilling, No Weeding, No Kidding!* Rodale Books, 2004. Detailed focus on layered gardening techniques for herbs.

Stout, Ruth. *The Ruth Stout No-Work Garden Book*. Bantam Books, 1973. Reprinted articles about straw bale and other lazy garden techniques.

Nature's Pest Control

❧ by Janice Sharkey ❧

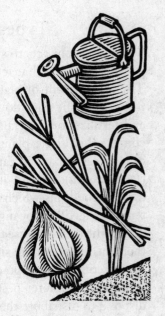

Plants are interesting entities. Apart from their floral beauty, scent, and edibility, many plants contain chemical compounds that help as natural deterrents against bacteria and viruses. As gardeners we can tap into the healing properties of certain herbs by using these chemicals in the battle against pests. However, before you begin concocting elaborate pest-control schemes, take a step back and mull over the old saying, "Know thy enemy." We must remember that sometimes the most obvious solution is to just allow the plant to grow healthy.

One way to help combat pests attacking your tender plants is to ensure they are given the best chance to be healthy and fight disease. Feed your plant from the soil upward, giving it the nutrients it needs, such as fertile compost, manure, or seaweed extract, and allow ample water and light for them to grow.

Grow Your Own Pest Deterrents

Cultivate herbs as natural remedies that you can harvest nearly year-round—such as rosemary, peppermint, and basil—by growing indoors, outdoors, and/or under glass. There is no substitute for fresh, young leaves picked that morning because they will retain more healing qualities than old or store-bought herbs. Besides, growing your own is far more economical and ecologically friendly.

Nature's Army

Attract beneficial insects to eat your pests by drawing them into your garden with biodiverse planting. Know what they want and provide tempting colors, flowers, scents, and particular plants—for instance, bees love coriander.

Types of Pest Control

Scent in a plant acts to attract natural pollinators, but it can also give off an aroma that acts as a barrier to pests that attack a plant. The lovely scent of plants that perfume the night air isn't just for our benefit, they do so for very practical reasons: protection and fertilization. Certain plants come under attack at night; to combat this, some plants emit a scented chemical that attracts other insects that will eat the predator, for example, moonflower (*Ipomoea alba*). Others, like pelargonium (the geranium family), have scented oils which deter pests. Some plants, such as nicotiana, are fertilized by night larvae insects and their scent is strongest in the dark because they have to attract insects like moths via their scent rather than sight, usually over a longer distance.

Of course, it's impractical to plant dozens of flowers in your garden just to deter pests. However, many options are at your disposal to distribute the right scent to protect your crops.

1. Scatter the scent by chopping up leaves of certain herbs whose leaves will give off a deterrent aroma sure to turn the pests away. Try using French marigolds to deter nematode worms or aphids from carrots.

2. Sprays are used as insect deterrents, to banish fungi and mildew, or to encourage growth. Unless otherwise stated, use four to eight drops of essential oil in four liters of water for spraying onto flowers, fruit, and vegetables.

3. Hanging strips of material from a stick or a branch with one drop of the proper neat essential oil on it can replace spraying. This is particularly useful when hung from branches of trees and it saves the arduous task of spraying such a large area. Renew when the scent fades or dries up.

4. Companion planting: One way to win the war against pests is to deter, confuse, and distract them from devouring your plants by growing certain "companion" plants as neighbors, which act as protectors. Thyme and lavender are marvelous at protecting all vegetables in the patch so plant them near kitchen gardens or use their oil in the watering can. Basil is an old favorite, which grows well with tomatoes because its scent deters aphids from attacking the tomatoes. Garlic is excellent grown next to roses. Peppermint is an undervalued herb that wards off all sorts of insects, including the cabbage-white butterfly (but do contain it in a pot, otherwise mint of any kind can be invasive).

Plant Chemistry

Each plant has its own protective medicine against its enemies, which are antibacterial and antiviral properties in its chemistry. We can extract these essential oils and use them on the whole garden. There are various ways to extract these oils: cutting up the leaf; squeezing the juice from fruit such as lemon or using the zest by grating the skin; using infused leaves to make an herbal tea; or simply harvesting and hanging up a bunch of drying herbs in the air. Once extracted, we can add the herbal oils to watering cans and sprays and apply around the garden. We can add essential oil neat to a bowl set out in the sun, which will stimulate the aroma to circulate and deter certain pests, such as midges.

Ingenious Foils

There are all sorts of green ways to deter unwelcome visitors to our gardens without resorting to undue expense or harmful chemicals. Often it can involve recycling "junk," such as cutting up plastic bottles and pushing them into the ground around a seedling. Later, the plant can be watered through the open hole at the top.

Cabbages can be protected from the larvae of the cabbage-white butterfly by wrapping tinfoil around their stalks or covering with enviro-mesh—a man-made barrier. Carrot flies hate mothballs, which can be crumbled up and scattered around on the soil. It is also good sense to plant before May and after June, thus avoiding the main activity period of the carrot fly.

Wasps can be made to do damage to themselves if you simply fill unwashed jam jars with water and hang them up, especially around fruit trees. The wasps suddenly turn into kamikaze pilots and dive-bomb into the jars, where, of course, they drown! Similarly, slugs are attracted to the beer-in-a-bowl trick, which can be an old margarine tub buried level to the ground. Slugs also have an acute sense of smell and hate garlic in any shape or form. Because garlic essential oil is so aromatically powerful, it can be rather unpleasant to handle. An easier option may be to break a garlic bulb into its cloves and place these in the ground, especially along the garden's edges where slugs often lay their eggs. French gardeners use crushed garlic: add one tablespoon to a watering can, mix well, and water the areas where the slugs are causing their damage. You can also protect the plants that attract the slugs—usually the thickest and most succulent plants you have—by laying a protective barrier of pine needles or holly around them. Save the needles from your Christmas tree to be ready for the war on slugs next summer. Any substance that is prickly or abrasive (such as eggshells or grit) will stand a good chance as an anti-slug carpet, as those annoying gastropods hate getting their tummies scored and will take their slimy selves elsewhere.

Know Your Enemy

Whether you plan to frustrate or destroy that pest, you need to understand what your dealing with. You can only succeed in thwarting them when you know what they are after and how they are likely to attack. Then you can devise a suitable plan for success. For instance, if birds are a problem in your garden, the strong color of lavender or violets planted near soft fruits can deter them. Using nets or crisscrossed colored string also keeps birds away from the fruit, which becomes more attractive as it ripens.

Natural Insect Repellents

Summer and autumn can be a nightmare in the garden, especially in the evening as various insects plague your outdoor living space. An ant invasion can be prevented by growing spearmint, tansy, or peppermint nearby. Citronella is another oil that is a natural insect repellent and can be put on cotton-wool balls and placed by doors. Aphids hate nasturtium, stinging nettle, garlic, basil, and resourceful parsley, so make room in your patch for these. Weevils get into pots and can destroy a plant quickly, so stick a clove of garlic in the pot to send them packing.

Making Plant Tea

Making herbal teas is a gentle way to transport the "active oils" of an herb to another plant. The tea plant should be harvested in the early morning before the sun evaporates the essential oils and prior to the plant flowering. Use one cup of fresh herb to two cups of water. Boil the water, pour onto the herbs and let it infuse for four hours or more. Strain off liquid and store. Use two tablespoons of this tea diluted in four liters of water in a watering-can or garden spray. Ideal choices would be peppermint or garlic to ward off aphids.

Enjoy Your Pest-Free Garden

Herbal oils not only control pests and make your crop stronger, better tasting, and more fragrant, they will also make your own time in the garden much more enjoyable. Mosquitoes have an aversion to the aroma of lemongrass, citronella, and lavender oils, (among others) and their use in the garden can take the sting out of hot summer nights. But all flying insects are a nuisance in the garden, especially if you are having a barbecue. The answer again is lemongrass or citronella essential oil, which may be used in several different ways. Add three drops to a bowl of water and soak some ribbons in this before attaching them to the branches of trees. You need to pay particular attention to clearing the areas under the trees and over water, as flying insects, including gnats and midges, love lurking around there. The pond can be cleared by putting some of the soaked ribbons on a pole and sticking this in the middle. Or you might find it easier and prettier to put a couple of neat drops of lemongrass or citronella on to an artificial flower or water lily and float that on the pond. If you have candles or flares outside, simply drop the essential oil onto the wax at the top, just as it begins to melt. If you have an outside light, put one drop of essential oil onto the bulb before you turn it on, and as the bulb heats up, the aroma molecules will be released into the immediate area and the flying insects will decide that there must be better places to hang out. If your summer evenings are being spoiled by moths, use the same procedures with lavender oil, which they hate.

By extracting the natural preventive medicine stored in herbs you can keep pests at bay. It's your choice whether to simply frustrate or annihilate them, but whatever method you adopt, using an herbal cure against garden pests is kinder to the ecosystem and your purse.

The American Mandrake

☙ by Ember ❧

Mandrake is a plant of many ominous legends and has a history of being associated with witchcraft—but it is native to Europe and not often easy to find. Yet many folks still seek out such plants for their gardens. While we may not have real mandrake (*Mandragora officinarum*) growing in our backyards in the United States, we do have an amazing plant often referred to as the 'American Mandrake.' Like mandrake, this unrelated plant, the May apple, is steeped in folklore, has some medicinal uses, and is dangerously toxic.

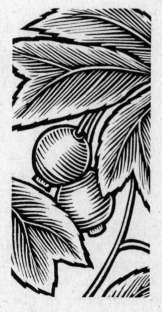

You may have seen May apple in the woods near your home, as it can be found in the eastern United States and Canada. (The umbrella-like leaves are hard to miss). Like a miniature forest, these "umbrellas" rise from single stems and can grow up to twelve inches wide and up to two feet tall. The attractive flowers, which appear in midspring, are pale yellow to white and have six to nine petals. They are usually turned down and hidden by the leaves, and are not fragrant. Though they don't contain nectar, the flowers are rich in pollen and are frequently visited by bumblebees and other insects. Each flower produces a fleshy, lemon-shaped berry sometime in May, which usually ripens in late summer or fall. This fruit is at first green, later turning yellow, is about two inches across, and possesses a strong scent. After the fruit matures, the leaves fall, and only the stems and fruit remain after summer.

May apple (*Podophyllum peltatum*) is a member of the barberry family and is native to North America, but it's a member of a tiny genus of plants probably originating in Asia. Its takes its name from the Greek: *podo*, meaning "foot" and *phylum*, meaning "leaf." *Peltatum* means "shield-shaped," so it appears there was some indecision on how best to name this plant. The deeply lobed leaves resemble both; and the name may be short for Anapodophyllum—*ana* referring to "duck" since the leaf also resembles the foot of a duck. Other common folk names include: vegetable calomel, Devil's apple, raccoon berry, ground apple, umbrella plant, Indian apple, hog apple, wild jalop, wild lemon, ground lemon, and Puck's foot.

May apple grows in colonies from a shared root system that spreads over great areas, creating miniature forests that can contain over a thousand stems. Each colony can be considered a single plant since each is genetically identical. The colony spreads about four feet per year, with new shoots appearing each year from a shared rhizome (horizontal underground stem). However, a colony must be twelve years old to flower and produce fruit. It takes a seed five years to form a rhizome, and seven more years for rhizome to make flowering stem. Seedlings rarely survive; new colonies are most often formed by animals that eat the fruit and deposit the seeds. The seeds seem to germinate better after being passed through the digestive tract of animals—and box turtles have been reported to have the highest success rate for transporting the seeds. Other animals enjoy the fruit, too, including raccoons and birds.

Not for Human Consumption

For humans, the fruit is edible only if it is ripe. It is toxic until then, just like every other part of the plant, including the seeds, and can cause diarrhea, severe gastroenteritis, and vomiting. But if the seeds are removed from the ripe fruit, the flesh has been noted for use in flavoring lemonade and making marmalade and jelly. However, most sources advise that these fruits should be consumed in moderation or avoided completely.

Ironically it is the rhizome, the most poisonous part of the May apple, that is the source of the plant's healing properties. Early American settlers used an extract from the root to ease constipation. The extract of the root is a "cathartic" (strong laxative) and has also been used for intestinal worms. This practice is discouraged, however, due to the risky nature of the plant's poison. The rhizomes were dried and ground into powder to eat or drink or to create a poultice for skin growths, especially warts.

This plant is reputed to have been used by the American Indians to treat many ailments, including snakebites. They also used it to induce vomiting and sweating and cure "skin cancer." Some tribes, notably the Menominees and Iroquois, even used May apple to kill potato bugs and corn worms. Sadly, it has been documented that they also used May apple to commit suicide.

Beginning in the 1970s and 1980s, the chemical containing the healing properties, podophyllotoxin, was tried as an anticancer agent, but proved too toxic. However, this led to other drugs, etoposide and teniposide, which block the division of diseased cells, and are semisynthetic, made by modifying compounds found in the plant. Studies have shown that a resin produced from the May apple proved effective on genital warts—which may have been the "skin cancer" the Native Americans referred to. Explorations are underway for treatment of rheumatism as

CLINTON PUBLIC LIBRARY
CLINTON, IOWA
52732

well. But even though extracts are being used for some skin cancers and genital warts today, self-medication should not be attempted. The plant is far too toxic and is rated unsafe by the Food and Drug Administration.

May apple is an attractive plant that can make a decorative addition to your own garden, if you wish. It makes an interesting ground cover and is best in slightly acidic soil. Transplants from root divisions can take place in summer, but take care not to remove plants from small colonies—and, as always, never take plants from protected areas or private property. Seeds can be removed from the ripe fruit and planted in early fall, but be careful where you plant them, as they can be quite invasive and choke out more tender plants. And, of course, use extreme caution if you have children around. One of the names for this plant, Devil's apple, came into use because children were told the plant was tended by the Devil in order to keep them away from it.

May apple in America suffers from habitat destruction and harvesting due to the new interest in medical uses. Studies are being made now to cultivate a variety of May apple that will produce more podophyllotoxin, which could result in a profitable agricultural crop. For its beauty, history, and medicinal uses, our 'American Mandrake' is a plant to be celebrated.

For Further Reading

Sanders, Jack. *The Secrets of Wildflowers*. The Lyons Press, Guilford, CT, 2003.

Swerdlow, Joel L. *Nature's Medicine: Plants that Heal*. National Geographic Society, Washington D.C., 2000.

Wilson, Craig. "May Apple." *Missouri Conservationist Magazine*, April, 1993.

Healing Weeds: Dandelion and Violet

❧ by Michelle Skye ❧

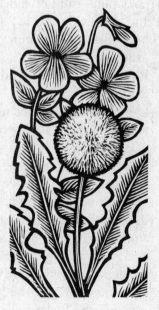

Who hasn't walked outside their door on a glorious, fresh spring morning and noticed the sweet, bobbing heads of the violet flower and the bright, predatory colors and spiky leaves of the dandelion? These two flowers bloom throughout the world and, often, are aggressively attacked by herbicides in order to achieve the movie-perfect, golf-course-green lawn. Yet dandelion and violet have been used for centuries for a variety of ailments. From headaches to insomnia, from digestive distress to poor liver function, these herbs aid our bodies with their plentiful vitamins and nutrients. Taking a close look at their beneficial properties may cause you to reassess their importance on your lawn and in your life.

Dandelion

The dandelion is a pugnacious flower that simply won't go away. Its root is thick and hearty, so unearthing it takes time and patience. Its flowers blossom into a brilliant yellow before dissolving into soft, seed puffballs. The puffballs allow the seeds to be picked up by airy breezes, scattering them throughout your neighborhood, up to five miles from the source! Dandelion's botanical name (*Taraxacum officinale*) comes from the Greek words for "disorder" and "remedy," causing some herbalists to speculate that the plant originated in Greece. Now, dandelion can be found all over the world, from China to Costa Rica to the United States. It is even cultivated in China, France, and Germany! Whether arriving on cue or showing up unexpectedly, this is a plant that loves to travel, packing healing medicine in its suitcases and valises.

Dandelion is a wonderful tonic herb with high levels of potassium, iron, calcium, ascorbic acid (a vitamin C complex), and vitamins A and B. As a diuretic, it supplies potassium to the body instead of draining it, speeding the healing of kidney and urinary problems. It can aid in alleviating fluid retention from PMS (premenstrual syndrome) and urine retention due to bladder infections. Dandelion's diuretic properties are also helpful in losing weight by reducing the water in the body and in regulating blood sugar by supporting the function of the liver.

Liver support is a major component of dandelion's medicinal package. The root of the dandelion aids in cleansing the liver by stimulating bile production. Bile is natural, bitter fluid secreted by the liver and stored in the gallbladder. Released into the duodenum (beginning section of the small intestine, near the stomach), it helps break down and digest fats in your body. Bile also helps transport toxins out of your body via stools. Thus, dandelion is a mild laxative that eases the removal of unnecessary elements from your body without causing diarrhea. Dandelion is wonderful for people with a slow or sluggish liver because of excessive alcohol consumption or poor diet. Besides serving as a restorative for the liver, it aids in preventing the formation of gallstones. (People with gallstones should avoid dandelion, however, as the herb could aggravate the condition.)

As a bitter, dandelion not only works with the liver and urinary tract, but also with the stomach. The leaves increase hydrochloric acid in your stomach, aiding in digestion and getting calcium out of your food. These help to increase the appetite of the elderly and those undergoing radical treatment, such as chemotherapy. Dandelion leaves can even lower your cholesterol! The leaves, like the roots, boost liver and urinary functions, but also work for bruises, fevers, and chronic skin problems like eczema, rashes, and acne. For these, you can utilize dandelion internally and topically, creating a poultice to put on the skin irritation.

Dandelion flowers also work on the skin, adding verve and zest. Worried about wrinkles, freckles, large pores, or oily skin? Create a flower infusion with the bright yellow dandelion flowers and splash it on your face in place of your regular skin toner. This is especially helpful for oily skin, but may be too strong for dry skin types. Despite their beautification abilities, dandelion flowers are not vain and insubstantial. Oh no! They are more than skin-deep, working below the surface to help alleviate depression, backaches, stomachaches, and menstrual cramps. Dandelion-flower oil can ease tension and aches in muscles, as well as in arthritic joints. The Flower Essence Society considers dandelion-flower oil to be helpful in the release of emotions locked in the muscles. This ability, in turn, promotes deep relaxation. So the next time you're giving or receiving a healing massage, try adding a few drops of dandelion to your regular massage oil.

Fiery and dynamic, the dandelion is an herb of many abilities and usages. You can create an oil, a poultice, or an infusion for use on the skin. You can drink it as a tincture or a tea (another word for infusion). Or (my personal favorite) you can go out and gather the leaves and blossoms right off the earth, for inclusion in salads, as tasty fried fritters, or in crafting dandelion wine. The possibilities are endless, as are the recipes!

Violet

Small and unobtrusive, thriving in the shade, along the edge of forest paths, down where the waters flow, violet is best recognized by full, heart-shaped leaves that start out rolled inward and unfurl with time. Violet, as the name implies, is often a deep purple but also can be found in shades of lavender, white, and pink—sometimes even on the same patch of earth. Growing in both wild and cultivated areas, it bridges the gap between city and country, wild witch and gardener. Such annual, early spring favorites as pansies and Johnny-jump-ups are violet varieties that possess many of the healing qualities of their wild cousins.

The bright, colorful violet flowers that decorate our doorsteps and hanging pots and forest glades are wonderful to eat as they are filled with delectably sweet honey that melts on the tongue. These violet flowers are simply for show, as they bloom too early for the honeybee to collect their honey and they house no seeds. So eat as many of them as you can gather!

The working flowers of the violet bloom in autumn. They are tiny and plain compared to their garish spring sisters, blending into the greenery with no petals and no scent, but with an abundance of seeds. The technical biological term for these types of plants is cleistogamous and they are self-fertilizing. Another way that these herbs reproduce is by sending out runners or scions from the main plant every summer after flowering. These scions, in turn, send out roots and become new plants, without the need of seeds of any kind.

With its powerful fertility, is it any wonder that violet gently strengthens and nourishes the reproductive system, along with the immune, respiratory, and digestive and urinary systems? Violet contains large amounts of vitamin A and ascorbic acid, a component of vitamin C. Like dandelion, violet assists digestion by allowing higher amounts of nutrients to be accepted into the body. And violet's powers have been known for centuries. Esteemed classical writers as Homer and Virgil sang its praises in verse.

The leaf of the violet is the most important and most medicinal part of the plant. In ancient herbal literature from the East and in scientific studies as recent as 1900, violet was shown to aid in the dissolution and healing of cancer, especially breast and skin cancer. (Ancient texts also claim that violet works in removing reproductive cancers as well, possibly because of the genital shape of the leaves.) With its high salicylic acid content, violet is especially useful with external cancers where compresses and violet water can be placed directly on the tumor. Drinking violet-infused water can also help to lessen and even remove lumps and cysts in the breasts. Some herbalists create violet breast-massage oil specifically for this purpose. Both the oil and the infusion can work to combat the monthly breast ache that often accompanies menstruation.

Violet continues her healing work with repair to wounds, sores, and swellings. Creating a poultice of violet leaves allows violet's antiseptic qualities to cleanse and repair the damage, cooling down the inflamed area. It is especially helpful for burns and boils—and even as a gargle for cold sores and cuts inside and around the mouth.

As a syrup, violet is best known for quieting sticky, thick, mucus-filled coughs, even whooping cough. She soothes sore throats and helps with difficult breathing due to congestion and colds. Utilizing both leaves and flowers, the syrup is gentle enough to give to children and not only helps with breathing, but relaxes and eases the little ones into a dreamy sleep. And for the adults who race about our crazy world, violet syrup is great for insomnia due to an overactive mind. A violet leaf infusion can supplement the syrup by easing tension headaches, anxiety, and restlessness.

A note of caution: Most recipes for violets utilize only the flowers and leaves of the plant. Violet roots, when eaten in large quantities, are toxic. You might consider using the roots externally, in poultices, to ease foot soreness or infection.

Violet's sweet presence lifts the spirits and brings out the smile in everyone. Consider making candied violets for your next party and using the flowers to decorate cakes or cookies. Eat them raw, right off the plant, or add violet leaves to your favorite spring salad (along with your dandelion leaves). Craft a violet oil or syrup or infusion and use them every day. You won't be sorry that you allowed the soft healing power of violet into your life!

Whether accustomed to herbal work or just starting out on the green path of healing, dandelion and violet are a wonderful and easy way to bring the healthful benefits of herbs into your life. Simple to locate, abundant and flourishing, dandelions and violets can be found all around the world . . . even in your backyard! So, next time you decide to mow the lawn, take a few moments to really look at the plants growing there. Perhaps you've overlooked a wondrous bounty of nutrition that has been provided for you by Mother Earth herself!

Herbal Pharmacy Terms

Decoction: an infusion that has been reduced to one-half of its volume due to evaporation

Infusion: a tea that has been steeped for a long time, usually utilizing much more herbal material

Oil (infused): a heated carrier oil (such as olive, almond, or jojoba) in which herbs have been steeped

Poultice: fresh or infused plant material that has been macerated and then placed on the skin. (A compress is a poultice that has been placed inside a cloth and then laid on the skin.)

Syrup: a decoction to which honey or sugar has been added

The Noble Bay

✺ by Susanna Reppert ✺

Then in my lavender I'll lay,
Muscado put along with it,
And here and there a leaf of bay,
Which still shall run along it.
  The Muses' Elysium,
  Michael Drayton, 1630

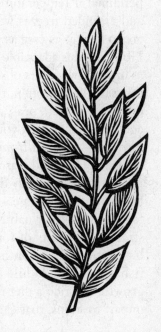

The noble Bay, *Laurus nobilis*, is native to Mediterranean shores and will not tolerate cold climates. On the other hand, it is a dandy houseplant and easy to grow into tubful proportions. The glossy evergreen leaves are both useful and decorative, which is why bay was selected the 2009 Herb of the Year by the International Herb Association.

For centuries, bay leaves have been used in cooking, garnishes, and as a symbol of victory, triumph, honor, and glory. As English herbalist John Parkinson wrote in the seventeenth century, "It serves to adorn the house of God, as well as of man; to procure warmth, comfort, and strength to the limmes of men and women by bathings and anoyntings out, and by drinks, etc. inward; to season the vessels wherein are preserved our meates, as well as our drinks, so drown or encircle as with a garland the heads of the living, and to sticke and decke forth the bodies of the dead." That covers just about everything.

Bay in the Garden

The bay tree is a favorite tub plant for terraces, driveway entrances, apartment houses, and restaurants, but it must be brought in during severe weather. Bay trees make magnificent houseplants that survive on just a shrug. Quite popular for topiary work, bay trees lend themselves to decorative pruning into oval, globular, conical, and standard shapes. Where winters are mild, this handsome evergreen is grown outdoors and can be sheared into a hedge. While the bay can handle first frosts, it's considered a tender perennial if temperatures drop below 25 degrees Fahrenheit—and extended freezes would kill it. Ideal conditions for the bay are to keep it as cool as possible, with generous amounts of sun. However, this adaptable plant will survive warm sills and tolerate as little as two hours of sunlight daily in the winter. If watering is occasionally forgotten, the negligence is forgiven. However, bay does best in rich, peaty, barely moist soil and loves good drainage. You may harvest your own bay leaves for cooking or making a wreath—plucked from the plant, the leaves bear little resemblance to the pallid seasoning at the supermarket.

Placed outside in the garden over the summer, the small bay plant will become a tree in several years reaching six to ten feet high. In their natural Mediterranean habitat, bay trees can stretch to heights of forty feet or more. The houseplant does best with a light monthly fertilizing with compost or a diluted fish emulsion. While generous feedings will inspire good growth, too rich a diet reduces the flavor and aroma that leaves impart to soups, roasts, and stews.

Bay is susceptible to scale and occasionally mealy bugs, but washing the leaves periodically with soapy water will keep it free of insects. Once you have noticed the pests, alcohol dabbed onto the leaves with cotton is the best remedy. Include all the leaf surfaces and stems in the treatment.

Bay is frequently confused with these other plants: the West Indian plant, *Myricia acria*, where bay rum cologne is from; or bayberry, *Myrica cerifera*, which is used for making fragrant soap and candles. Laurel, *Kalmia latifolia*, the state flower of Pennsylvania, is handsome in the landscape and poisonous to ingest. To compound the confusion further are other casual references to California Laurel, *Umbellularia californica*. This is bay's benign sibling and the only other species of Laurus. A native to the Canary Islands, it is less hardy than bay, with longer, broader, and less tasty leaves. While these plants are each interesting unto themselves, their differences are botanical as well as in their usefulness. The similarity lies in the uses of the words *bay* or *laurel* and also the fact that each has handsome, glossy, fragrant leaves.

As you can see, the names bay and laurel have been given to many plants down through the centuries. Unless you are the proud possessor of a true bay tree, confine your culinary flavorings to the dried bay leaves purchased from any reputable spice company. Do not experiment with these other botanicals, no matter how similar the name, appearance, or fragrance. On the other hand, do not cook without the noble bay.

Bay in the Kitchen

In the kitchen, a cook can have a good time showing off culinary talents by using bay leaves. They are used in marinades and are one of the main ingredients in the classic "bouquet garni" of French cooking. Bay is also a common ingredient in pickling spices and these leaves were a favorite standby for flavoring custards and puddings in England.

Bay's strong flavor should be used sparingly. Crumble half a bay leaf in a can of consommé or vegetable soup to make the flavor sparkle, or drop a leaf into your favorite stew, casserole dish, or spaghetti recipes: Here is one of my favorite recipes:

Spaghetti Sauce

1	green pepper
1	large onion
4	stalks celery
2	cloves garlic
4	tablespoons olive oil
2	cups tomato sauce
1	teaspoon basil
½	teaspoon thyme
1	whole bay leaf
1	whole clove
6	sprigs parsley
1	tablespoon oregano
1	teaspoon crushed rosemary
1	tablespoon salt
2	cans tomato paste

Dice the green pepper, onion, celery, and garlic, then brown lightly in the oil. Add all remaining herbs, tomato sauce, and tomato paste and simmer slowly for several hours until thick.

For an elegant touch, use handsome leaves from your bay tree as a garnish for your roasts and favorite dinners served on a platter. This was a tradition in merry olde England.

The leathery foliage of bay leaves does not soften in the soup, sauce, or stew pot and are not easily chewed or swallowed. Because the leaves are easy to catch in the throat and possibly choke on, you should remove the whole bay leaf before serving your meal. In our family, if you're lucky enough to get the bay leaf in your bowl, you win! And get to do the dishes!

The French have an easy way to add and subtract the bay leaf—the bouquet garni, a bunch of herbs tied together and lowered into the stew pot with a long string. Dried herbs can be put into squares of cheesecloth and used the same way.

Bouquet Garni

12	whole bay leaves
12	teaspoons whole celery seeds
24	whole cloves
36	peppercorns
12	tablespoons dried parsley
6	teaspoons dried thyme

Divide the ingredients equally onto twelve, 4-inch square pieces of muslin or cheesecloth. Tie with heavy white twine, leaving a long string attached for easy removal when done cooking.

Pantry Helper

Here is a household hint worth its weight in gold. Store large bay leaves, a dozen or so, in any container of starchy products such as pasta, rice, cornstarch, flour, cereal, or biscuit mix where they effectively repel weevils. Be sure to keep the leaves whole and to use lots of them. They will not influence the flavor of your food. Use these bay leaves in cooking and replace them in the canisters as necessary. If they are whole they will be easy to transfer from an empty container to your next full box. They are also valuable used in the same way with paprika, chili powder, and any other weevil-prone spices.

Multiple Uses for Bay

In aromatherapy, the steam-distilled essential oil derived from the bay leaves used in cooking has a wonderfully spicy aroma. Bay is an antibacterial oil, specifically recommended in a steam inhalation for tonsillitis or added to any cold and flu blend. Emotionally, the essential oil is both uplifting and grounding, helping to clear mental confusion and clarify thought processes. As such, it might be an effective addition to a study blend. However, the oil can cause skin sensitivity and should be used as a part of a blend and not directly on the skin.

Bay can be an interesting addition to hair care blends as it's said to stimulate hair growth and clear dandruff. To make a bay shampoo: gather 8 bay leaves, mix in ¼ cup chamomile and ¼ cup rosemary. Add the herbs to 1½ pints of boiling distilled water. Steep for 10 minutes. Add 1 pint of your favorite shampoo to this infusion.

Bay has a grand history, and is often carried at funerals, weddings and state occasions. The bay of history and poetry is the bay passed into Greek mythology by the legend of the nymph Daphne, who was loved and pursued by Apollo. Daphne fled from his amorous advances and was changed into a bay tree. Thence it became sacred to Apollo, and since he was the god of poetry, it followed that the traditional bay wreath was presented as an award to university graduates in rhetoric and poetry, the most notable of whom became poet laureate, crowned with bay laurel. Ancient Greeks crowned not only scholars, but also Olympic winners with bay wreaths.

An easy bay leaf wreath can be made by poking 16-inch gauge wire through bay leaves, dried cinnamon sticks, and dried orange pieces. Shape the wire into a wreath as you go. Simply twist the two ends of the wire together with pliers and add a raffia tie for the bow and "ta-da!" you have a lovely bay leaf kitchen wreath.

This just scratches the surface of the creative uses for the heralded bay. As Thomas Lupton eloquently pointed out in his 1575 publication, *Book of Notable Things*, "Neither Witch or devil, thunder or lightning will hurt man in the place where a bay tree is."

All this and it repels weevils too!

Grasses in the Herb Garden

❧ by James Kambos ❧

Grass is the most widespread herb in the world. From the tropics to the arctic, grasses flourish. Many herbalists tend to ignore grasses when planning an herb garden, but grass is perhaps the most important herb known to humankind.

With every breath we take, we should be grateful for grass. Grass can sometimes be plain and modest in appearance, but it is a life-giving plant. Along with trees, the grasses purify and add oxygen to the air we breathe.

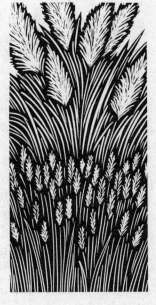

Grasses have also been raised as food crops since ancient times. Oats, wheat, barley, corn, sugar cane, and sorghum are some of the great grasses used as food, which helped fuel civilization. Once grasses were domesticated, the human race shifted from a nomadic hunting/gathering lifestyle to a settled agrarian society. After the ancients learned they could plant and harvest these grasses, the human race became partners with nature rather than only taking from it. This was the beginning of agriculture, one of the most significant events in human history.

Perhaps the first vegetation to emerge on Earth was grass, and over the ages its appearance has changed very little.

Today the grass family contains about five thousand species. These include everything from a single blade of grass that has taken root in cracked pavement to a Midwestern corn field ripening beneath the August sun. It also includes the ornamental grasses, which you can use in the herb garden.

Using Grasses in The Herb Garden

Most herb gardeners have enough space to include one or two varieties of grass in their gardens. Depending on the ultimate size of the grass you select, grasses could be used as an edging or ground cover, or a larger variety such as the eight-foot tall Pampas grass could serve as a dramatic focal point.

There are many aesthetic reasons to add grass to the herb garden. Grasses add texture, grace, and refinement—imagine slender blades of grass swaying gently in the slightest breeze on a summer day, with the flower heads silhouetted against the sunlight.

With the many grass selections available, grass can also add color to the garden. Foliage colors can range from green, blue, gold, burgundy, to almost white. The foliage may also be solid or variegated.

Instead of traditional flowers, grass produces plumes or spikes in shades such as rose, cream, and gold. These spikes are prized for their use in herbal crafts such as wreaths and other dried arrangements.

If left on the plant, the plumes and spikes will add a softness and texture to the herb garden that few plants can achieve.

The Vanishing Grasslands of North America

There was a time when the magnificent grasslands and prairies of North America stretched from western Ohio to east of the Rocky Mountains, and from Oklahoma north into Canada. This was the most vast grassland in the world. It was home to the buffalo herds that grazed upon the grasses.

Growing among the grasses were beautiful wildflowers with charming names—evening primrose, Indian paintbrush, and blazing star to name a few. Sadly, much of the virgin prairies have been destroyed; only sections remain. Luckily, some of these are now protected. The grasslands are part of our national heritage and serve as habitats for beneficial insects, birds, and butterflies.

By incorporating a few ornamental grasses suitable to your geographic area into your herb garden, you can help recreate the grassland habitat in a small way. Perhaps if more people were aware of the importance of grasses during the early twentieth century, the devastating Dust Bowl of the 1930s wouldn't have occurred. So, adding grasses to the herb garden can also benefit the environment.

A Selection of Grasses

There are more than forty varieties of grasses available to the home gardener today, ranging in size from eight feet tall to a diminutive eight inches tall. You'll find varieties suitable for wet or dry soils.

What follows is a group of grasses suitable for a wide range of growing conditions including some native American species; all are nondemanding and easy to grow. Any of the following plants are worthy additions to even the most refined herb garden.

Northern Sea Oats (*Chasmanthium Latifolium*): This native grass will remind you of a day at the shore. It grows to three feet, is easy to grow in sun or shade, and isn't fussy about soil or moisture. Both stems and seed heads are wheat-colored. It looks charming in a cottage garden.

Silver Pampas Grass (*Cortaderia Selloana*): Among the most dramatic of all grasses, this handsome plant will form a four-foot-wide clump. The stems rise to eight feet under favorable conditions and are topped by creamy white flower heads, which reach their peak in late summer. Plant as a specimen or team up with butterfly bush for a contrast in color and texture.

Blue Fescue (*Festuca*): Growing to only eight to ten inches in height, this fescue is perfect to use as an edging, ground cover, or in the rock garden. The foliage is dusty blue and spiky. It likes sun and dry soil. This small grass can make a big statement when planted in groups among rocks leading down a slope to a pond. Blue fescue also looks smashing planted in front of a cream- or terra cotta-colored stucco wall.

Gold Hakone Grass (*Hakonechloa Macra*) 'All Gold': This is an elegant shade-tolerant grass which reaches about twelve inches high and eighteen inches wide. The foliage has a cascading habit and forms a lovely clump. I have two of these grasses nestled among ferns and hostas where their gold foliage brightens a shady corner of my herb garden. The lightest breeze stirs its slender blades, which adds to this plant's appeal. It never becomes invasive.

Red Wind Hakone Grass (*Hakonechloa Macra*)'Beni-Kaze': A grass that was first featured on the market in 2007 is also fond of shade. Ultimate size is two feet by two feet. The slender foliage is green, but it takes on shades of red as autumn approaches. Red Wind is ideal planted at the edge of the border where its foliage creates a soft transition from lawn to herb bed.

Switch Grass (*Panicum Virgatum*): When the wagon trains moved westward it's very possible the settlers saw this grass. At one time, this native prairie grass grew on the North American plains. Fortunately, this grass can still be purchased at garden centers. It is extremely tolerant of wet or dry soils and grows in full to partial sun. Mature height is four feet; width, two feet. The upright foliage is green and burgundy at the same time, turning all burgundy in the fall. I planted this grass along with other prairie plants such as coneflower (echinacea), which is a very pleasing combination. Late summer brings attractive seed heads. It's versatile and carefree.

Rose Fountain Grass (*Pennisetum Alopecuroides*): The stems are slender and green, but by midsummer the entire plant is covered with showy, fuzzy, pink flower heads that you can't keep from touching. An average plant grows three feet high and wide in average soil. It's ideal in the middle of the herb border, where its arching habit adds a graceful touch. The flower heads dry quickly, giving you a wealth of craft material.

Bluestem Grass (*Schizachyrium Scoparium*): Tough and drought tolerant, Bluestem will perform well in any soil if given full sun. Bluestem grass is another native prairie grass. The leaves can be a blue/purple shade and are topped with cream or silver seed heads. Overall height is two to three feet. Autumn turns the plant to a rich russet color. An easy grower, Bluestem brings a bit of the American prairie to the herb garden.

These are only a few of the grasses on the market today suitable for the herb garden. I've mentioned them because I've personally handled them and have found them to be long-lived. Check with local nurseries, master gardeners, or your county extension agent to see what grasses are adaptable to your area.

Maintenance

Grasses are among the easiest herbs to grow. Providing you select a grass suitable for the planting site you're landscaping, a grass plant is usually carefree. But, here are some tips:

Don't overfertilize. For most grasses, average soil is usually all that's required.

Let the grass plant die back naturally in the fall. This will add visual interest to the garden during the winter, and the plant will be able to catch and sculpt the falling snow. Besides that, the sound of the wind rustling through the dried stems on a cold blustery day is pure magic.

When you see new growth appearing at the base of the plant in early spring, cut the dead growth back to just above the emerging stems.

Companion Plants

Grass can be stunning planted alone or with several clumps of the same variety grouped together. Here are some beauty ideas.

To create a meadow habitat similar to the American prairie, mix some wildflowers with your grasses. Coreopsis, liatris (blazing star), black-eyed Susan, gaillardia, and coneflower are good choices. All coneflowers—purple, white, and gold—are at home when planted in a grassland theme.

Another idea is to combine grass with plants that share a similar growth habit. For example, daylilies with their arching foliage planted with grass would create a garden with an appealing form, and give the border a unified look. Liriope with its grasslike foliage would give a similar effect. Or for an elegant look, try grouping the blue-stemmed grasses with silvery-green herbs like lavender, sage, and wormwood.

Keep Our Earth Green

Before human or beast walked on this Earth grasses were growing wild and untamed. And they were already ancient.

Your front yard or a city park aren't just attractive green spaces, they provide us with life-giving oxygen. If not for grass, life on our planet as we know it wouldn't exist.

Over the centuries we have abused and even tried to destroy grass. This happened in part due to overgrazing and poor land management (remember the Dust Bowl). But still, it endures.

When you add an ornamental grass to the herb garden you're not only making an investment in beauty, you're also helping keep our planet green.

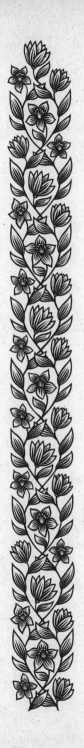

Culinary
Herbs

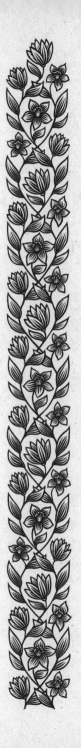

Practical Pestos

❧ by Suzanne Ress ❧

Most everybody is fond of classic basil pesto sauce on pasta—it could be considered one of Italy's more recent contributions to internationally popular cuisine. The first published recipe for basil pesto as we know it was in the Ratto brothers' Genoese cooking manual in 1865, though the brothers didn't invent pesto sauce. No one really knows who did, but we do know it has been around a very long time. It was even mentioned in Virgil's "Bucolique," written about 30 BC. Pesto is probably the oldest oil-based sauce known; millennia older than mayonnaise!

The herb basil, known as the "royal herb," was imported to Europe from Asia Minor in Roman times, and took to the mild climate and soil of the Italian Liguria and neighboring French Provence regions like dandelions to a

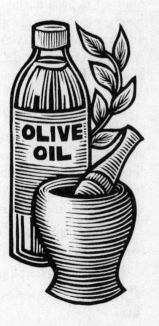

summer lawn. Liguria (where Genoa is) is known as the birthplace of pesto, and Provence as the home of the very similar French pistou basil sauce. Originally, because basil doesn't dry well, making pesto was a way to enjoy the full flavor of basil all year long. The olive oil works as a preservative for the herb's essential oils and bright green color. Pine nuts and cheese were added as binding agents to give the sauce a thicker consistency, and adding garlic brought out the herb's unique sweet peppery flavor.

Traditionally, Genoese basil pesto is made in a marble mortar, using a wooden pestle. While I won't argue with the pesto purists, I have found a small electric food processor to be more efficient, and it makes perfectly delicious pestos.

The word *pesto* in Italian means crushed, beaten, or stamped upon—quite violent sounding! Here in northern Italy, small signs on well-kept strips of lawn warn us not to "crush the herbal carpet"—a polite way of saying "keep off the grass." When reading such a sign, because of the wording in Italian, I think of my feet crushing the grass into pesto sauce. And, in fact, why restrict yourself to basil in the making of pesto sauce? My experiments have yet to include lawn grass pesto, but I have found that almost any fresh herb (or combination of herbs) can be employed in making wonderfully delectable pesto sauces to be eaten on or in anything from soup to ice cream!

Green Goddess Mixed Herb Pesto Dip

For starters, try this smoothly exciting light green dip. In this, and most of my pesto recipes, I only use half a garlic clove when the garlic is very fresh and big in late spring and summer. In winter, a whole clove or two could be necessary. Because this recipe contains cream cheese as a binding agent, nuts are not needed.

½–2   garlic cloves

½   lemon, juiced

Parsley, a small handful

10   basil leaves

       3   lovage leaves
       4   savory stems, 3 inches long
       3   oregano stems, 5 inches long
       ¼   cup olive oil
       8   ounces cream cheese, softened
       ¼   cup parmesan, grated

Cut the garlic into 3 or 4 pieces and toss these into a small food processor with the juice of ½ lemon. Blend well. Rinse and tear the leaf herbs into pieces, remove the stems from the savory and oregano, and toss the herbs into the machine. Run slowly until finely minced. Pour the olive oil slowly into the processor as it is going, and increase the speed to emulsify. Add a tablespoon of the cream cheese and blend again, until mixture is smooth and green. Transfer mixture into a glass bowl, and stir in the grated parmesan and the rest of the cream cheese. Chill. Serve with plain salted potato chips and celery sticks.

Chive and Fennel Pesto for Bruschette

These tasty treats are easy to make, crunchy, garlicky, and pretty on a serving plate, making them great as an appetizer, side dish, or party food.

    ¼–1   clove garlic
       2   tablespoons unsalted pistachios (or pine nuts),
             shelled
           Chives, a small bunch
           Fennel flowers, leaves, and tender stems, a handful
       ¼   cup olive oil
       ¼   cup pecorino cheese, grated
      12   small slices whole wheat or French bread
       6   cherry tomatoes
      12   pitted black olives

Cut the garlic into several pieces and toss it in the processor with the fresh unsalted green pistachios (or pine nuts). Blend well. Add rinsed and cut chives and fennel. Blend until the herbs are finely minced. With machine still running, slowly add the oil and increase speed to emulsify. Transfer the mixture into a small bowl and stir in the grated pecorino. Always stir in (don't mix in processor) grated hard cheeses, as it gives the pesto a better texture.

Toast the bread slices directly on the rack in a 400-degree F. oven (not in a toaster—they won't be as crunchy!) While still warm, spread a generous amount of pesto on each toast slice, then top with half a cherry tomato and a pitted black olive. Arrange slices on a serving platter and enjoy!

Salad Dressing Pesto

Nasturtium leaf is peppery and blends well with the cool fresh flavor of borage leaf and celery-like pungency of ajwain. This dressing works well on a freshly picked and made up green salad of lolla rossa, rucola, and valerian leaves. Decorate with pretty blue borage flowers and bright red and yellow nasturtium blossoms—all edible!

½–1 garlic clove

6 shelled walnuts, halved

10 nasturtium leaves

4 borage leaves

8 ajwain, 2-inch fronds

3 tablespoons olive oil

2 tablespoons fizzy water

½ lemon

Cut garlic into several pieces and toss into processor with walnut halves. Blend well. Rinse and tear herbs into bite-sized pieces and put into processor. Process slowly until herbs are finely minced. Slowly add oil and increase speed to emulsify. Add

2 tablespoons fizzy water and blend until very smooth. Squeeze in a few drops of lemon juice and add salt and pepper to taste. Just before serving salad, pour dressing over all and toss well.

Vegetable Soup with Pesto

Similar to French Pistou, this delicious summer vegetable soup is intensified by the addition of the mixed-herb pesto.

Soup

16	ounces plum tomatoes, canned
2	potatoes
2	carrots
1	zucchini
1	shallot
4	cups vegetable broth
12	ounces white beans, canned
½	cup tiny pasta

Pesto

1	garlic clove
2	tablespoons pine nuts
16	basil leaves
2	4-inch stems oregano
2	leaves Russian sage
10	sprigs parsley
2	3-inch stems thyme
¼	cup olive oil
¼	cup parmesan, grated

First, start the soup. Empty the can of tomatoes into a large cooking pot, and crush them a bit with a potato masher. Set this on a medium heat and add the potatoes, carrots, zucchini, and shallot, all cut into bite-sized pieces. Let it simmer about 10 minutes while you are making the pesto.

For the pesto: Cut the garlic clove into pieces and put it and the pine nuts into the food processor and blend well. Add the rinsed and torn up herbs (tough stems removed) and blend until herbs are minced. Slowly add the oil and increase speed to emulsify. Place this in a small bowl and stir in the grated Parmesan.

Now, back to the soup: Add the broth and the canned beans, and bring it back to a simmer. Add the pasta and cook for a few more minutes, according to package instructions. When done, ladle soup into serving bowls, plop a big tablespoon full of the pesto into the center of each bowl, and serve. The pesto is then stirred into the soup before eating. (Serves 4)

Eggs and Asparagus with Tarragon Pesto

This dish makes a nice light supper for late spring when the asparagus are fresh and the tarragon tender and flavorful.

1	garlic clove
2	tablespoons pine nuts
	tarragon, a fistful
15	small leaves lemon balm
¼	cup olive oil
2	tablespoons Parmesan, grated
8	slices whole wheat or sourdough bread
	Butter
½	pound asparagus, trimmed
8	eggs

Make the pesto first: Process garlic with pine nuts, add rinsed and trimmed herbs, and blend until finely minced. Slowly add oil and emulsify. Transfer to a small bowl and stir in grated Parmesan cheese.

Now put 1½ inches of water into two large shallow pans with lids, and place them on high heat to come to a boil while you toast and butter the bread slices. Arrange the buttered toast slices, two on each plate. Place the trimmed asparagus into one of the pans, put the lid on, and turn down the flame to medium. After 3 minutes, poach the eggs in the other pan. After 4 more minutes, turn off the asparagus, take one ladle of the hot asparagus water and stir it into the pesto, then drain the rest. Place 4 or 5 asparagus spears on each slice of toast. Slide a poached egg on top of each asparagus "bed." Drizzle a generous tablespoon of pesto over each egg and serve. (Serves 4)

Shiso Pesto for Pumpkin-Filled Tortellini

If you can't find pumpkin-filled tortellini, you can substitute the ones with spinach and ricotta, or even plain cheese, filling.

2	tablespoons pine nuts
	Chives, a fistful
12	shiso leaves
6	calendula flowers, petals
¼	cup olive oil
2	tablespoons pecorino, grated
1	tablespoon Parmesan, grated
1	pound pumpkin-filled tortellini, packaged fresh

First make the pesto. Process the pine nuts. Add the rinsed and cut chives, the torn shiso leaves, and only the petals of the calendula flowers. Blend until well minced. Slowly add olive oil and continue blending until the mixture is very smooth. Transfer to a small bowl and stir in the grated cheeses.

Cook the tortellini according to package directions. Just before draining, add 1 or 2 spoonfuls of the hot cooking water to the pesto. Drain tortellini, place in a large bowl, pour the pesto over all, stir well, and serve. Mild and soothing! (Serves 4)

Five-Herb Pesto Risotto

Pesto

2 tablespoons walnuts

4 sprigs parsley

2 basil leaves

3 6-inch stems marjoram

2 4-inch stems savory

10 shiso leaves

¼ cup olive oil

2 tablespoons (each) pecorino and Parmesan, grated

Risotto

2 tablespoons olive oil

2 garlic cloves, chopped

1 onion, chopped

2 cups arborio rice

2 tablespoons pine nuts

1 cup dry white wine

1–3 cups vegetable broth

For the pesto: Process the walnuts. Add the rinsed and trimmed herbs and process until finely minced. Slowly add olive oil and emulsify. Place in a small bowl and stir in grated cheeses.

For the risotto: Heat 2 tablespoons olive oil in a large pot over medium high heat. Add chopped garlic and onion and sauté until transparent. Add rice and pine nuts and let toast a few minutes, then add 1 cup white wine. Pour a glass for yourself as you continue cooking (optional). Stir the rice, and when wine is absorbed, add the broth, one cup at a time, adding more as the previous one becomes absorbed into the rice. Cook for about 18 minutes total. When the risotto is done, turn off the heat, stir in the pesto, mix well, and serve. (Serves 4)

Pesto Rub for Baked or Grilled Chicken

The oil and herbs in the pesto keep the meat moist and tender.

2	tablespoons unsalted green pistachios
½–1	clove garlic, diced
3	2-inch stems lemon thyme
8	3-inch stems marjoram
3	small, young bay leaves
¼	cup olive oil
1	shallot, chopped
1	tablespoon white wine
	Salt and pepper
3	pounds chicken pieces

Process the pistachios with the cut up garlic. Remove the thyme and marjoram leaves from their tough stems, and add these to the pistachios, with the small, fresh bay leaves. Process until finely minced. Slowly add olive oil and emulsify. Transfer to a small bowl and stir in finely chopped shallot and white wine, then salt and pepper to taste.

Using your hands, rub each piece of chicken all over with the pesto, and then leave the chicken pieces in a covered container in the refrigerator for an hour. Bake 30 to 45 minutes at 350 degrees F., or grill until done. (Serves 4)

Spicy Pesto Rub for Grilled Steak

½	clove garlic
¼	teaspoon lemon zest
10	5-inch stems hyssop
6	2-inch stems savory
½–1	red pepper
2	tablespoons olive oil

2   tablespoons Cognac

2   1-inch thick tender steaks
        (i.e. marbled beef entrecote, a rib steak)

Process the garlic and lemon zest together. Add rinsed and trimmed herbs and red pepper (minus its seeds!). Process until finely minced. Add olive oil and emulsify. Add cognac. Blend until very smooth.

Using your hands, rub pesto all over both sides of each steak. Place in a covered container and refrigerate for an hour. Remove from refrigerator 15 to 20 minutes before placing on the hot grill. Grill and salt to taste. Enjoy these steaks with plenty of fresh bread, sliced juicy red tomatoes, and a favorite bottle of dry red wine. (Serves 2)

Dill and Chive Pesto for Salmon

½   clove garlic

2   tablespoons pine nuts

5   4-inch fronds of dill

    Chives, a fistful

2   lemon verbena leaves

¼   cup olive oil

4   salmon steaks

To make the pesto, process the garlic with the pine nuts until well blended. Cut the dill fronds and chives with scissors, and tear the lemon verbena leaves into pieces. Add these to the garlic and nuts in the processor. Blend again until the herbs are finely minced. Slowly add the oil, and increase processing speed to emulsify.

Using a table knife, spread a thin layer of pesto over one side of each salmon steak. Cook, nonpesto side down, on a medium grill or in a 400-degree F. oven for 10 to 12 minutes. (Serves 4)

Roast Vegetables with Pesto

4 yellow onions, cut into eighths

8 potatoes, peeled and cut into 1-inch cubes

12 ounces fresh green beans, cleaned, and cut into 1-inch pieces

Salt and pepper

For the Pesto

½ clove garlic

6 walnut halves

1 5-inch stem rosemary

3 3-inch stems thyme

1 sage leaf, large

¼ cup olive oil

2 tablespoons Parmesan, grated

2 tablespoons pecorino

2 tablespoons dry white wine

Preheat oven to 350 degrees F. Oil a large rectangular pan and put in prepared onions, potatoes, and green beans. Add salt and pepper and stir well. Roast for 45 minutes, stirring after 20 minutes. In the meantime, prepare the pesto.

Process garlic with walnuts until well blended. Remove tough stems from rosemary and thyme and put the rest, with the torn up sage leaf, into the processor, and mince well.

Slowly add ¼ cup oil and emulsify. When mixture is quite smooth, transfer it to a small bowl. Stir in grated cheeses. Add 2 tablespoons of wine and stir. When vegetables are done, pour pesto over everything, mix well, and serve. (Serves 4)

Sweet Pesto Ice Cream

Don't tell anyone this ice cream contains almost no sugar. They will never guess that the stevia makes it so sweet.

4–5	stevia leaves, large
18	lemon balm leaves
15	peppermint leaves
3	rose geranium leaves
1	lemon verbena leaf
½	lime
1	pound fresh mascarpone cheese
1	cup whipping cream
1	teaspoon vanilla
1–3	tablespoons powdered sugar

Rinse and tear all the leaves into pieces and process slowly with the juice of ½ lime until the herbs are finely minced. Add 2 tablespoons of the mascarpone and process until no leaf particles are visible. It will seem coagulated, but it's OK. Transfer mixture to a freezer-proof container and stir in the rest of the mascarpone. Put it, uncovered, into freezer.

Whip the cream, add vanilla and powdered sugar, and refrigerate. After 1 to 2 hours, take mascarpone/herb mixture out of freezer and process in large food processor until smooth.

Fold in the whipped cream. Freeze another 2 to 3 hours. Serve with thin dark chocolate wafer cookies. Very refreshing! Store covered.

These are a few of my own herb pesto recipes, but I often improvise according to what herbs are in season or in need of a "trim." Feel free to experiment and use the herbs you have at hand to create new taste combinations.

At the end of the growing season one of the many nice ways to use up herbs is to make larger quantities of several different kinds of pesto to be frozen in useful amounts, in labeled plastic freezer bags. During the cold winter months, the lively flavors of homemade herbal pestos will continue to arouse the taste buds of you and your loved ones.

Winter and Summer Savory

≫ by Anne Sala ≪

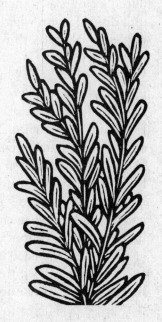

S imilar in flavor and use, yet different in habit, summer and winter savory are perfect subjects for a Victorian-like literary device: the allegory. They are sisters raised apart from each other under very different conditions. Winter savory toiled in the hot lands of the Mediterranean where her growth was stunted, while summer savory grew wild and leggy in the mountains of Eastern Europe. It is only when they are reunited and their peppery personalities compared side by side that anyone can tell that the two herbs are related. One savory is often mistaken for the other in flavor, but each shines in her own way.

Winter savory (*Satureia montana*) is a shrublike perennial from the Mediterranean with semi-evergreen leaves. It is an important herb in the

Provence region of France and the Acadian communities of North America.

Summer savory (*Satureia hortensis*) is a sprawling annual with tender leaves that grows easily from seed. It is reputed to originate in Eurasia and is an important ingredient in many cuisines from the Balkan area.

Savory's botanical name, *Satureia*, is said to come from the herb's ancient association with satyrs, the mythic half-man, half-goat creatures with an insatiable sexual appetite. Satyrs were said to live in fields of summer savory, and their lustiness sprang from the plant's pungent scent. This association makes it a popular element in love potions. Conversely, winter savory has gained a reputation as a libido suppressant.

Both savories have been used in seasoning mixes since ancient times because their flavor is so powerful. It has a hot bite mixed with the taste of thyme, mint, and lemon, which added a contrasting component to food before black pepper was introduced from Asia. Some word historians say the herb's influence on a dish's flavor is where we get the term "savory" foods, meaning particularly flavorful in a rich—usually not sweet—way.

Winter savory is a cornerstone of the classic herb mixture, "herbes de Provence." In France, it is sometimes called *poivrette*, meaning "little pepper."

The Romans carried summer savory with them as they expanded their empire. They infused vinegar with it and used it as a wholesale condiment. When the Pilgrims sailed to the New World, they brought along summer savory to remind them of their gardens in England.

Both savories are common ingredients in recipes for slow-cooked and cured meats, such as salami. Unfortunately, the herbs have fallen out of favor in American kitchens and gardens, and are rarely included in modern recipes.

Nevertheless, winter and summer savory remain important ingredients in many European cuisines to this day. For instance,

Bulgarians still place dried summer savory on the table alongside salt and pepper to season their dinner.

The Germans call savory bohenkraut, meaning "bean herb." Summer savory's flavor marries well with green beans, and winter savory is a great addition to the pot when boiling dried beans. Both herbs are said to have gas-reducing properties and are a good general tonic for the digestive track.

When hunting for a recipe that uses winter or summer savory, many simply call for "savory." One would think that meant the two are interchangeable, but not really. Ask anyone from Bulgaria or France, and they will insist that the savory from their area has the strongest flavor and the most medicinal benefits.

Depending on the personal tastes of the recipe's author, they often suggest one savory and discount the other. It seems best, however, to use the type that is common to the country where the recipe originates. Failing that, use summer savory for dishes that are prepared quickly, or when the savory will be eaten fresh. Use winter savory when the recipe calls for a long cook time so the leaves have a chance to break down.

Play around with adding the herb to recipes that need a little more depth. Include summer savory leaves in salads. Put a pinch of winter savory in the saucepan when poaching pears.

Green Beans and Summer Savory

Let's start with a simple recipe. Adding a sprig or two of summer savory to the boiling water completely infuses the beans with the herb's flavor.

 1 pound trimmed young green beans

 1 tablespoon chopped fresh summer savory
   (or ½ teaspoon dried)

 2 2-inch sprigs fresh summer savory
   (or a pinch dried)

 2 tablespoons butter

   Salt and pepper to taste

1. Bring a pot of water to a boil with the sprigs or pinch of summer savory.

2. Drop in the green beans and cook on high heat, uncovered for about 6 minutes until tender and bright green.

3. Drain the beans and return to the pot.

4. Lower the heat under the pot and add the butter and chopped savory to the beans.

5. Stir occasionally for about 1 minute, until all butter melts.

6. Serve with salt and pepper. (Serves 4)

Herbes de Provence

Bay leaves lose their flavor quickly when they are ground into a powder. This is probably why it has become difficult to find bay powder in stores. Look online if you do not have luck in your local grocery stores. For the sake of experience, I ground my own with my mortar and pestle, just to see what it was like. It took about 100 bay leaves and about 5 hours of hard grinding to make a tablespoon. Next time, I'll order online.

Purists claim that basil should not be an ingredient in herbes de Provence. Others, including some from the Provence region, believe it is an acceptable addition since the herb has become so common in Mediterranean food. I left it out of this recipe so the winter savory could have a more pronounced influence, but feel free to add 1 tablespoon of dried basil to this mixture.

1   teaspoon fennel seed

1   tablespoon powdered bay leaves

2   tablespoons dried winter savory leaves

1½   tablespoons dried sage leaves

1½   tablespoons dried thyme leaves

1½   tablespoons dried rosemary leaves

1   teaspoon dried Greek oregano

2   teaspoons dried lavender buds

1. Crush the fennel with a mortar and pestle or food processor. Place in a bowl and add the powdered bay leaves.

2. Gently break down remaining ingredients, except for lavender, with a mortar and pestle or food processor. You just want the pieces to get a little smaller, not turn into powder. Mix with fennel and bay leaves.

3. Add lavender buds, either whole or crushed.

4. Mix all the ingredients and store in an airtight jar. It will keep for several months. (Recipe makes about a half cup)

Pork Loin Chops with Herbes de Provence in Red Wine Reduction

This is one of my favorite dinners when I don't have a lot of time. Serve with corn and rice boiled in broth.

1	tablespoon olive oil
1	tablespoon herbes de Provence
½	teaspoon salt
2	tablespoons flour
4	boneless pork loin chops (about 1 to 1½ pounds)
¾	cup red wine

1. Place a 12-inch skillet over medium-high heat. Film the bottom with the olive oil.

2. Combine herbes de Provence, salt, and flour on a plate and spread out.

3. Dredge each chop in the flour mixture, shaking off the excess. Place each one in the hot pan and lightly sear for about a minute on each side. A crust does not need to form.

4. Add the red wine to the skillet and let it bubble briskly until it has nearly all boiled off. Occasionally flip the chops so they take on a purple hue. This should take about 10 minutes.

5. Serve the chops immediately, using the wine reduction as a sauce. (Serves 4)

Roast Chicken with Winter Savory
en Papillote

Cooking meats and vegetables in paper parcels is popular in France. It makes the meat exceptionally tender. Carrots have an affinity for savory, so they make a nice accompaniment to this dish. Serve with rice or mashed potatoes, to soak up the juices.

It is possible to prepare the chicken in a baking dish, without the paper, but the unusual packaging makes for a dramatic presentation at the dinner table.

8	2½-foot sheets of parchment paper
4–6	3-inch sprigs of fresh winter savory, rinsed and dried
1½	teaspoons salt (less if using salted butter)
1	teaspoon ground black pepper
1¼	sticks butter, softened
1	3½ to 4½ pound chicken, cut into 4 to 6 parts, skin on (do not use wings)
6–8	carrots (about 2 cups), peeled and cut into ¼-inch discs

1. Put two sheets of parchment paper together and fold in half so all four cut edges are lined up. Starting at the folded edge, cut out the largest half heart shape you can (yes, just like you were taught in grade school). Repeat with the remaining sheets of parchment paper.

2. Preheat oven to 350 degrees F.

3. Remove winter savory leaves from the stems and place leaves in a bowl with the salt and pepper.

4. Take one stick of softened, but not liquefied, butter. Combine with winter savory, salt and pepper.

5. With the help of a small, sharp knife, lift the skin of each chicken piece from the meat to create a pocket. Be careful not

to separate the skin entirely from the piece. Use your hands to slather the butter mixture on the meat under the skin. This is messy; it is perfectly acceptable to get butter on the outside of the skin.

6. Place the chicken piece in the center of a lobe of the double-stacked, heart-shaped papers, close to—but not too near—the crease. Surround it with ½ cup carrots. Pull over the other half of the heart, so the two sheets fall loosely over the contents. Begin to fold over the edges of a short section of the paper near the divot at the top of the heart. Crease the fold firmly with your fingers, and then fold it again. While maintaining the double-fold with one hand, begin to fold over the next bit of paper, so the two folded sections overlap. Repeat this procedure until you have double-folded the entire edge and come to the heart's point. Twist the point tightly to hold the folds in place. Repeat with the remaining parchment sheets, chicken pieces, and carrots.

7. Place the parcels on a baking sheet.

8. Melt the remaining ½ stick of butter. Brush it on the top of the parcels.

9. Bake for 30 to 40 minutes. Chicken should be cooked to an internal temperature of 180 degrees F. You may want to sacrifice the beauty of your own parcel to check, if such things worry you.

10. Transfer each parcel to a dinner plate. Set before your guests and instruct them to carefully tear into the paper with their dinner knives. Watch out for the steam! (Serves 4)

Roasted Pineapple with Summer Savory

To truly appreciate this sweet-tart dessert, I encourage you to begin with whole pineapples—or at least ones that have been cored for you at your local market. Canned pineapple might be too juicy.

2 pineapples, peeled, cored, and
        sliced into 6 to 8 rounds each

¼ cup summer savory leaves, rinsed and dried

¼ cup brown sugar, plus more for sprinkling

½ stick butter

   Vanilla ice cream

1. Make sure the primary oven rack is not in the topmost position because you do not want the pineapples to scorch. Then preheat oven to 450 degrees F.

2. Place the pineapple rounds on a tinfoil-lined baking sheet. You may need to roast them in two batches.

3. First sprinkle summer savory leaves on the pineapple, then sprinkle with brown sugar. You do not need to completely blanket the slices.

4. Put the baking sheet in the oven for 5 to 8 minutes. The pineapple should look a little dry, but not burned.

5. Melt the butter and mix with the brown sugar.

6. Brush the pineapple with the butter and sugar mixture.

7. Cook for another 10 minutes. The pineapples should start to caramelize and even begin to deflate.

8. If baking the pineapple in two batches, remove the first batch and use a spatula or fork to remove the gooey rounds from the tinfoil before they start to stick, and set on a plate. Tent the plate with tinfoil to keep warm.

9. Repeat steps for the second batch.

10. Scoop ice cream into bowls, top with pineapple rounds. (Serves 4)

For Further Reading

Gardiner, Anthony *Herbes de Provence: Seven Top Provençal Chefs and Their Recipes*. Trafalgar Square Publishing, 2002.

Gardner, Jo Ann. *Living with Herbs: A Treasury of Useful Plants for the Home and Garden*. The Countryman Press, 1997.

What's Cooking?
Check out the
Goddesses' Kitchens

⤳ by Nancy V. Bennett ⤳

It's 5 pm and you are uninspired and hungry. A quick wander through your pantry will turn up the usual, and sooner than you can say "frozen cardboard," you're heading for one of those prepackaged foods. Hang on a minute! In the goddesses' kitchen, we can find foods not only to tempt our tummies, but also turn on our minds, if only we take a moment to look at their history.

Start your meal off with Eperona Bachiques, or "The Spurs of Bacchus," another name for a spicy shrimp appetizer. Follow it with Ceres' Bounty Bread. Add in a dish of tortellini, or as the Italians call it, the *Umbilichi Sacri* or the "goddess's navels," inspired by a late night Venus. Finish it off with a fabulous dessert or drink inspired by Minthe. You have a feast fit for, well,

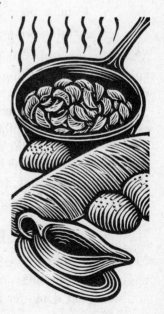

you know. These recipes are fun, fast, and easy, so why settle for a TV dinner?

An Appetizer from Bacchus

Bacchus was the god of wine and overindulgence. He also had to be fast on his heels with all that dancing and womanizing! For those who prefer their shrimp unwrapped, this recipe can also be made without the bacon.

Spicy Spurs of Bacchus

5	strips of bacon, halved
10	jumbo shrimp, thawed, deveined, and shelled
1	tablespoon ground thyme
1	tablespoon ground oregano
1	tablespoon cumin
1	tablespoon ground white pepper
1	tablespoon chili powder
2	tablespoons paprika

Make the most of your time the night before by pre-cooking your bacon and shelling/deveining the shrimp (or buy it prepared). Store covered in the refrigerator.

Take the strips of bacon and cook until limp, not crispy. Set aside to cool. Then combine the spices in a bowl. Evenly coat the 10 jumbo shrimp in the spices. Wrap bacon around the shrimp and secure with toothpicks. Fry in a pan until bacon is crispy and shrimp are bright pink. It is good paired with a nice cold beer or a chilled glass of Riesling wine.

Break Bread with Ceres

Ceres was the goddess of agriculture, who taught us mere mortals how to grow and store our own crops. She was also a mother, and when her daughter Persephone was snatched away by the god of the underworld, she made the world "fall" into a cold and dying time.

This is how the ancients explained the changing of the seasons, for Persephone is with her mother for half the year and with her husband for the other. Ceres never forgave that nasty Pluto (Hades) for taking her little girl. And you thought you had problems with your in-laws! This simple-to-put-together recipe is for those busy days in honor of protective mothers everywhere.

Ceres' Bounty Bread

Now, you don't expect me to make you bake tonight as well? Instead, buy a loaf of fresh French bread. Whole wheat French bread is even better. Keep a presliced loaf in the freezer (cut horizontally down the center). For the spread, the following combination works well:

½ cup softened butter

1 teaspoon fresh parsley

1 teaspoon fresh tarragon

1 teaspoon fresh chives

Mix the chopped herbs into the butter until evenly distributed. You can experiment with combinations of your favorite herbs, but probably shouldn't exceed 3 teaspoons total per ½ cup of butter. Spread generously on the bread and wrap in foil.

In a preheated oven (350 degrees F.) let the bread warm until butter is melted (about 20 minutes if thawed, 25 to 30 minutes if frozen). Serve with some goddess's navels (see next page), or nibble between courses.

Helpful hint No. 1: Herb butter is a great thing to have on hand. If you have time, make extra by doubling the recipe. Place excess butter on wax paper and roll it in a log, which can then be wrapped and stored in the freezer for later use. A pat or round of herbed butter makes a nice touch to fish, steamed vegetables, or pasta!

Helpful hint No. 2: You can also prebutter a loaf of French bread. Wrap and stick it in the freezer, ready for a fast snack or addition to a meal.

Venus' Navels

Long ago in the city of Bologna, Venus decided to spend a night at an inn near the outskirts of town. Of course her beauty did not go unnoticed, and the innkeeper decided to take a peek through the keyhole of her door while the goddess was undressing. All he got to see was her navel. But what a navel! Inspired by that beautiful belly button, he hurried to his kitchen to make the world's first tortellini, and the rest is culinary history.

Peeping Tom Pasta

For this recipe you can choose from either a fresh cheese tortellini (usually found in the refrigerated areas of grocery stores and often sold in 16-ounce packages) or a dried one. Prepare tortellini according to package instructions. Plan on cooking about 10 tortellini per serving. While it is cooking, make this wonderful herb sauce. **Hint:** If you precook the tortellini, you can drain it and set it aside with a little olive oil mixed in. Keep a pan of water just barely boiling, and plunge the tortellini in for a couple of minutes to warm, right before you serve.

Sauce

> 1½ cups almonds
>
> ½ cup pine nuts
>
> 3 tablespoons butter

Melt butter in a large frying pan. When butter is foamy, add the nuts. Stir often and let the nuts brown.

Add:

> 2 tablespoons fresh parsley, chopped
>
> 1 teaspoon fresh lemon thyme (or regular thyme), chopped

1   teaspoon fresh chives, chopped

2   teaspoons white flour (to thicken sauce)

Salt and pepper to taste. Mix well.

Add:

¼   cup ricotta cheese

¼   cup whipping cream

Stir until sauce has thickened, adjusting heat if needed. Remove from heat. Stir into the hot pasta and top with some chopped parsley and a sprinkle of nutmeg. Serve immediately.

A Trod Under Finish

To finish off your meal, you can choose from two minty offerings: a large portion of mint ice cream with chocolate sauce and a crumbled up brownie (you'll see why in the story) decorated with a few sprigs of fresh mint, or a cold traditional Southern drink called a mint julep. The first one, you can figure out for yourself. Below is a recipe for the drink, which is very refreshing, especially after a yummy meal. It is a make-ahead dish that is best started the night before and kept ready in the refrigerator.

Mint, or Minthe, by the way, was a saucy little nymph who caught the eye of the god Hades. It did not sit well with the other love of his life, Persephone, who caused the poor girl to be turned into dust after being trod upon by the jealous goddess, (hence the brownie crumbs!). Hades caused the mint plant to spring up from the dust, and it has been delighting our taste buds and noses ever since.

Mint Julep

2   cups water

2   cups white sugar

10   mint sprigs

2   ounces whiskey (or ginger ale)

Make a syrup by combining 2 cups water with 2 cups white sugar. Cool. Add 7 to 10 sprigs of mint and cover, letting the flavors combine overnight.

To prepare, take a cup of crushed ice and pour a tablespoon of the syrup over it. Add 2 ounces whiskey (for an alcoholic version) or ginger ale for a nonalcoholic version. Stir, and decorate with a sprig of mint. Put up your feet and relax.

Assess for the Future

Wasn't that easy? Don't you feel you deserve a good meal, being the domestic goddess that you are? Put away that frozen pizza and reach for some fresh herbs instead. Be inspired to make every meal a celebration for your senses.

The Herbal Loaf

⚘ by Kaaren Christ ⚘

Home-baked bread encourages deep breaths. It reminds us to savor each moment. As our loaves rise—once, twice, or even three times—we are reminded to travel a path of patience. Peeking under warm towels into the baker's bowl offers the delightful experience of anticipation. Even the yeasty scent of bread rising affects our emotions, reminding us of times we felt most loved and nurtured. Bread is about home and our connection with others.

We can shape the personality of our bread by choosing ingredients to add to the dough. We can also slather bread with a variety of spreads, both sweet and savory. Bakers around the world have always added seeds, dried and fresh fruit, and nuts to enhance the flavor of the bread. Each combination of ingredients subtly changes the

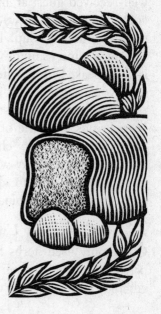

overall nature of the loaf. These changes are made even more exciting with the addition of fresh or dried herbs.

Quick bread is cousin to yeast bread, and also changes personality when herbs and other complementary ingredients are added. A quick bread is simply a bread made using baking soda or baking powder as the leavening agent instead of yeast. Most people are familiar with the most popular quick breads: banana, poppy seed, or pumpkin loaf. Quick breads, which also include scones, biscuits, and breads twists, may not always create the sentimental response that yeast bread elicits, but they have their own gifts. Quick breads save the day when unexpected company arrives and have an enticing aroma when fresh from the oven. They also keep well when wrapped tightly, and freeze well too. Just as with yeast breads, herbs can be added to quick bread to sweeten or make savory.

The Savory Loaf

The savory loaf—one seasoned with herbs, spices or salt—is a well-received guest at any lunch or dinner table. These loaves complement rich stews and casseroles and are a favorite for dunking into hot soup. The savory loaf is even more welcomed on a long winter's night when our desire for hearty, dense bread is at its peak. Whole wheat, rye, spelt, and pumpernickel flours are favorites during this time of year.

Herbs can be added to white, whole wheat, and mixed-grain yeast breads any time of the year in a variety of combinations. Herbs are specifically chosen to complement particular meals. With a little creativity while combining, herbs and spices allow us to create elegant breads we would expect to find only in fancy restaurants. The combinations are almost limitless!

Commonly Used Herbs for Savory Loaves

Commonly used herbs for the savory loaf include mint, basil, parsley, oregano, thyme, rosemary, tarragon, thyme, sage, chervil, marjoram, and savory.

There are also many other ingredients that work well together with fresh herbs. A few include garlic, onions and hot peppers such a jalapeno, or chilies. Sun-dried tomatoes, a wide variety of cheeses, and olives are also popular.

Herbs for Bread with Beef Stews, Stroganoffs, and Soups

Use gently sautéed onions and parsley in bread that will accompany homey beef dishes. Finely dice an onion and cook it over low heat until the onions are soft and translucent. Allow onions to cool while you are kneading the dough, and work them in just before you are finished. Dice fresh parsley and add as well. The use of onion and parsley in this manner complements any traditional beef dish.

For more sophisticated beef dishes boasting a generous amount of sherry, wine, or specialty mushrooms, consider the use of thyme. It works particularly well in a French bread, paired with fresh garlic. Tarragon is also associated with more elegant dishes. Both can be added raw before the last rising of the loaf. For variety, work different combinations of herbs and ingredients into an assortment of forms. Buns, individual loaves, or bread sticks are all options aside from the standard loaf.

For Fish, Fish Stews, and Bouillabaisses

Seafood has a more delicate flavor than beef, so bread accompanying it requires a gentler culinary approach. Choose herbs for your bread that will not smother the natural flavor of the seafood. If you are serving a sauce likely to be sopped up with a fresh slice of home-baked bread, this is even more important. White bread is the most common choice of bread to accompany fish because of its gentle, light texture and flavor.

Lemon is often used to complement seafood dishes. Mother Nature offers us a number of lemony herbs for our loaves, such as lemon basil, lemon thyme, and lemon verbena. Use lemon zest to speckle the bread with beautiful yellow flecks. For a different result, try fresh or dried dill, which works wonderfully with delicate white fish such as sole or halibut.

Lamb: If you are planning to serve bread with your perfect lamb dish, look no further than rosemary, oregano, or mint to complement the loaf. I would suggest sticking to one herb as opposed to combining. Each flavor stands well on its own.

Herbal French Bread

1	tablespoon active dry yeast
2	tablespoons honey
1	teaspoon salt
3½	cups unbleached flour
1	cup milk
1	tablespoon white vinegar
¼	cup water
6	tablespoons butter
½	cup minced onion
1	clove garlic, minced
½	teaspoon salt
1	tablespoon minced parsley
1	tablespoon tarragon
2	tablespoons oil

Combine yeast, honey, 1 teaspoon salt, and 1½ cups flour.

In a small separate pot, combine milk, water, and 4 tablespoons (¼ cup) of the butter; heat until warm. Add this milk mixture and vinegar to the flour mixture, then stir until blended.

Stir in 1½ cups additional flour to form sticky dough. Turn dough onto floured surface and knead well. Add enough flour to create a smooth dough. Place dough in a greased bowl and let rise until doubled in size.

Punch down dough and roll into a long rectangle on a floured board.

In a saucepan, heat the onion, garlic, salt, parsley, tarragon, and 2 tablespoons butter until butter is melted. Spread over the dough rectangle and starting from the long side of the rectangle, roll the dough into a tight tube.

Place the bread seam side down onto a greased cookie sheet and let rise until doubled in sized.

Preheat oven to 400 degrees F. Bake bread until golden brown, about 20 to 30 minutes. Brush hot bread with melted butter and sprinkle with chopped parsley.

Savory Spreads

If you prefer to keep your bread dough free of herbs but want to experiment with their flavors, try a savory spread. This way you can make a number of different herb spreads, adding them to only one slice at a time and deciding which flavors you enjoy. This also accommodates a number of dinner guests with different tastes.

The most common savory spread is garlic butter. Garlic butter typically includes butter, freshly crushed garlic, and fresh parsley. Garlic butter is a wonderful spread for French bread, which often accompanies pasta dishes. You can adjust the amount of garlic to suit your own taste.

But let's not stop at garlic! Combine 1 cup of softened butter with ⅓ cup of your chosen herb. Favorites for herbed butters are parsley, dill, and basil, but you can try any kind you like. Once well combined, let the mixture sit covered on the counter overnight so the flavor of the herb can permeate the butter fully. This butter can be used on almost any savory bread imaginable.

Infusions

You can also "infuse" a bread with an herb, which means that you saturate the dough before or after baking. Although less common, this technique works well with recipes for quick breads, such as this rosemary bread twist.

Rosemary Bread Twists

⅓   cup butter

2¼   cups whole wheat pastry flour

¾   teaspoon salt

2   tablespoons Parmesan cheese

3½   teaspoons baking powder

1   cup milk

1   teaspoon dried rosemary, crushed

1   teaspoon minced garlic

Preheat oven to 400 degrees F. Melt butter in a 9 × 13-inch baking pan. In a mixing bowl, combine flour, salt, cheese, and baking powder. Stir in milk until just mixed. On a floured board, knead bread until smooth. Roll it into a 12 × 6-inch rectangle. Cut into 12 strips (1 × 6 inches). Stir the rosemary and garlic into melted butter. Twist the strips of dough 6 times, then coat with melted butter. Bake for 20 to 25 minutes or until lightly browned.

The Sweeter Side of Bread

Sweet bread has a naturally "social" personality. They are favorites for celebrations and ceremonies like birthdays, seasonal celebrations, and anniversaries. They are also a favorite loaf to offer friends or family on special occasions—or for no occasion at all!

Sweet breads can be herbed according to season. In spring, try poppy seeds with lemon verbena and lemongrass; the result is as delightful and fresh as the season. When summer arrives and you want to be in the garden instead of the kitchen, turn to the quick bread. Scones, biscuits, and quick loaves can be enhanced with freshly chopped spearmint, peppermint, or rose petals. These herbs can be combined with stronger spices such as cinnamon or lemon. For even more seasonal flair, add summer fruits such as plums, peaches, raspberries, and blueberries to your quick bread.

When cooler weather comes, return to the pleasure of yeast breads and indulge in the heady spices of nutmeg (which can be ground as needed) and ginger (consider the use of candied or freshly ground ginger). As fresh herbs are a little harder to come by, you might consider freezing some herbs such as lemon verbena and lemon balm to use to sweeten your bread in the depths of winter.

Almond, Poppyseed, and Lemon Verbena Scones

2   cups all-purpose flour

⅓   cup sugar

1   tablespoon poppy seeds

1   teaspoon baking powder

½   teaspoon salt

½   cup vegetable shortening, chilled and cut into bits

¼   cup butter; unsalted, chilled and cut into bits

⅓   cup sour cream

1   large egg

2   teaspoons almond extract

4   tablespoons finely chopped lemon verbena

Preheat oven to 350 degrees F. Mix the first five ingredients in a food processor. Add the shortening and butter. Using on/off pulses, process until the mixture resembles coarse meal. Whisk sour cream, egg, almond extract, and lemon verbena in a small bowl to blend. Add to the flour mixture in the food processor and pulse just until dough forms ball. Transfer the dough to a lightly floured work surface and knead only enough to form a solid ball. Using hands, press into a 15 × 3-inch rectangle. Cut into six 3 × 2½-inch pieces and then cut each piece diagonally to form twelve triangles. Place the scones on a heavy baking sheet, spacing 1 inch apart. Bake until puffed and pale golden, about 15 minutes.

Herbal Honey

Herbal honey is a lovely way to sweeten a loaf and it's perfect for those who are hesitant to add things to favorite recipes. Favorite herbs to add to honey include delicately flavored rose petals, lavender, and peppermint.

To make, add 4 tablespoons of your chosen herb to one cup of honey. The mixture should then be placed into glass jars that have been sterilized in boiling water and left to air-dry thoroughly.

The Last Loaf

Although the flavor combinations are infinite, here are some of my favorites.

- Parsley, chives, and onion (savory)
- Oregano, basil, and sun-dried tomato (savory)
- Cinnamon, lemon zest, and lemon balm (sweet)
- Basil, carmelized onion, and cracked pepper (savory)
- Rosemary, chives, and parsley (savory)
- Dried apricot, almonds, and lavender (sweet)

Bread is such a wonderful part of our diet, in part because of the variety of ways we can alter its nature with herbs. There are literally thousands of ways to introduce fresh herbs directly into (or onto) your bread. Be adventurous! Try different kinds of flour, experiment with different forms, use complementary ingredients, and try both yeast and nonyeast breads. Any way you choose, you get the added benefit of the healthfulness of herbs.

Classic Herb Combos

≈ by Alice DeVille ≈

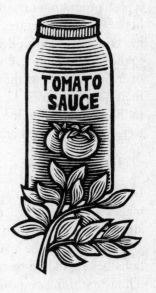

I grew up in a family that planted a garden of herbs and vegetables every year. No matter where we lived (we moved frequently before my teen years) or how small the plot of land, there was an abundant harvest. The savory dishes we enjoyed included fresh herbs that sat in water on the windowsill or were drying on paper towels and then in a warm oven before freezing or storing in jars for later use. Combined with home-canned fresh tomatoes, there is nothing as delicious as a simple, basil-infused tomato sauce to dress up an entree pasta, a bruschetta accompaniment, a hearty stew or a homemade Margherita-style pizza.

If you seldom use herbs or don't know where to find them, you needn't worry—it's easy to get started. A majority of cooks prefer dried herbs and stock their favorites in the pantry. They are easy to use and require little or no prep time before adding to recipes. For practical reasons, don't buy the larger sizes of dried herbs, especially if the ingredient is one you'll seldom use. They won't maintain their freshness and won't season the dish. If in doubt, smell the contents of the jar—no aroma means the herb is past its prime. Herbs are easy to buy at the local supermarket, usually located in the spice aisle alphabetically and by brand name. Subtle advertising attracts customers who are unsure how to use herbs. Specialty stores, outdoor markets, and cookware emporiums sell herbs and often place them strategically near foods, cookbooks open to specific recipes, and kitchen products.

Food preparation with fresh herbs has really caught on in the last decade. Thanks to The Food Network and The Public Broadcasting System, an infusion of cooking shows has introduced consumers to an even wider array of uses for herbs and spices. A typical program shows the cook going to the garden, picking fresh herbs, and chopping them to add to the recipe du jour. Or the chef has bouquets of fresh herbs in water readily accessible for adding to the featured recipe. Out of convenience, most of us buy bundles of fragrant herbs at the market to dress up favorite dishes with their delicate flavors. These herb packages typically last two weeks in the refrigerator as long as you don't wash them and store them wet—water rots the herb and leaves unsightly brown spots.

What Your Taste Buds Tell You

In many recipes, herbs take center stage. The quantity used makes all the difference in the recipe's outcome. Some herbs are more pungent than others. Fresh herbs reach their fullest aroma if you rub the leaves between your hands and cut into ribbons before adding to recipes. Use dried herbs more sparingly. The worst thing you can do is add too much of a dried herb to a recipe and overpower the dish beyond palatability. If you do make a mistake, add a peeled raw potato to the pot to absorb the pungency. It is OK to substitute dried herbs for fresh. The rule of thumb is to use three to five times more fresh herbs than dried, depending on the strength of the herb.

Develop the flavor of dried herbs by soaking them in a liquid for several minutes before adding them to your recipe. The "liquid" normally is a main ingredient of the dish such as stock, broth, lemon, oil, water, or vinegar. Play with either freshly chopped or dried herbs by working them with your hands before using them as a rub for meat, fish, or poultry. One of my favorite French dressings has parsley and basil mixed with lemon juice, olive oil, salt, and pepper. Before adding the other ingredients, I chop the herbs and place them in the oil for an hour to allow the flavor to emerge. By adding 2 tablespoons of Dijon mustard to this same recipe, you have an excellent marinade for fresh fish or grilled shrimp.

Serious French cooks use herbes de Provence to liven up a variety of recipes. Gift shops and grocery stores in France and elsewhere sell them in small cloth sacks to the delight of tourists. The typical mix includes savory, rosemary, marjoram, oregano, and thyme in variable proportion. This flavor enhancer can be used alone or mixed with other herbs. Bundles may be placed directly in soups, stews, or inside the cavity of poultry.

One of my favorite accompaniments to filet mignon or standing rib roast is a mushroom ragout made with three types of mushrooms and flavored with sprigs of fresh thyme, cream, unsalted butter, and Madeira wine. Even vegetarians ask for seconds, sans boeuf.

Maximizing the Flavor of Herbs in Recipes

You can do so much to save time when using herbs. If you don't think you can use all of the fresh herbs you buy or you grow your own herbs and don't want them to go to seed before you use them, try this tip. Dry them and freeze them in the combinations you use most. All you have to do is take a package out of the freezer and add it to the recipe's liquid and you're in business. Don't know the best combinations to freeze? Here are a few suggestions: basil, thyme, and Italian flat-leaf parsley; marjoram and thyme (excellent rub for meats and poultry or a vegetable dish topper); chives and dill weed (good with egg, fish, or cheese dishes); dill, mint, and parsley (wonderful for salad seasonings); sage, thyme, and chives (perfect for dips and fancy butters); and oregano, basil, and thyme (perk up tomato dishes, sauces, and soups).

Want to make flavored vinegars? Try combining sage, parsley, shallots, and red wine vinegar; chilies, garlic, oregano, and cider vinegar or fennel, garlic, parsley, and white wine vinegar. Flavor oils with these combinations: dill, garlic, and sunflower or canola oil; oregano, thyme, garlic, and olive oil; or chervil, tarragon, shallots, and peanut oil. Combine marjoram and garlic with butter for a savory treat. I put this combination in tiny butter molds and freeze them. Use them to top a serving of meat, chicken, or fish, place them on ice and serve with your favorite rolls at the dinner table or place the butter shapes on your buffet table to serve as one of the spreads for cocktail bread loaves.

Using herbs creatively helps you cut down on the use of salt. My recipe for cooking a 3-pound beef eye roast is absolutely delicious, yet its main seasonings are dried thyme and black pepper, which are added after the meat has been seared in oil and butter in a Dutch oven to seal in the juices. (Yes, I do use real butter, which contributes to the rich brown crust that makes the accompanying gravy a masterpiece.) After I add water and beef broth and other seasonings, the roast goes in the oven covered, and 90 minutes later, I add vegetables such as carrots, small white onions, and potatoes or leeks and cook for another hour. Although you can eat this dish right out of the pot, I make a savory gravy from the remaining liquid in the pot. Just remove the meat and vegetables to a rimmed platter, cover to keep warm and set meat juices. Then make a roué of butter, flour, and kosher salt (the only salt in this recipe). Remove from heat to prevent lumps, whisk in the juices (at least 2 cups), and return to low heat until mixture thickens.

Featured Recipes

The following eggplant recipe is one of my Italian favorites that I developed about ten years ago. This version is a meal in itself and works well with a green salad, crusty bread, and a glass of red wine. If you open a window while you're cooking it, the neighbors may be over for dinner.

Stuffed Eggplant

2   firm, medium-size purple eggplants
    (wash skin thoroughly)

1   medium onion, chopped

½   pound ground beef (optional, may
    be prepared meatless)

2   large cloves garlic, minced

2   zucchini, chopped in 1-inch chunks

2   yellow squash, chopped in 1-inch chunks

⅓   yellow or orange pepper, diced

⅓   green pepper, diced

2   tablespoons extra virgin olive oil
    (add more if necessary)

8   ounces canned tomato sauce (may substitute
    with canned petite diced tomatoes)

3–4 fresh Italian plum or Campari tomatoes chopped

8   large basil leaves, chopped in ribbons

¼   cup chopped Italian flat-leaf parsley

    Kosher salt and freshly ground black pepper,
    season to taste

1   medium Italian or French roll, crumbled

1   cup grated parmeggiano-reggiano cheese

Directions: Preheat oven to 350 degrees F. Cut off stem ends of eggplants. Cut eggplants in half lengthwise. Take a sharp paring knife and run it around the perimeter of each eggplant leaving ¼ inch of flesh. Scoop out pulp and cut into 1-inch cubes. Lightly salt and pepper the insides of the eggplant shells. Heat a 12-inch skillet on medium heat. When hot, add 2 tablespoons olive oil. Add chopped onion and ground beef and brown. Add garlic the last 2 minutes to avoid burning and stir. Next, add the chopped zucchini, yellow squash, and diced green and yellow pepper. Add salt and pepper. When the squashes have browned slightly, add the eggplant pulp and mix thoroughly. Season lightly. You may need another tablespoon of olive oil or more to prevent sticking.

Place the eggplant shells cut-side down over top of the browning vegetables to soften slightly. Remove shells to add next ingredients and cover again with shells. When the vegetables are browned but still firm, add the tomato sauce and stir. Add the chopped tomato, basil, and parsley. Stir in the crumbled roll until all ingredients are moist. Cook on low heat for 10 minutes. Then stir in half of the grated cheese and combine well. Taste to adjust seasoning. Place the eggplant shells in a 12 × 9-inch baking dish. Add the prepared stuffing. Sprinkle with remaining cheese and bake for 20 minutes. Serves 4 to 6.

You can also use this recipe for eggplant caponata by omitting the ground beef and adding a tablespoon of finely chopped capers. Then prepare according to directions. When the mixture cools, put into a blender or food processor and serve at room temperature with small bread rounds, crackers, or vegetables.

I adapted the following recipe from one that appeared in the food section of my utility company's monthly magazine. Here I'm using several fresh herbs. The blended flavors add excitement to the taste and make this dish perfect for healthy summer eating.

Mediterranean Chicken Salad

2 pounds boneless, skinless chicken breast

12 ounces Caesar dressing

1 red onion, cut in quarters

1 red pepper, cut in half and seeded
1 tablespoon garlic, chopped
1 tablespoon fresh chives, chopped
1 tablespoon fresh rosemary, chopped
1 tablespoon fresh parsley, chopped
1 tablespoon fresh thyme, chopped
1 tablespoon fresh oregano, chopped
8 ounces crumbled feta cheese or shredded
     fresh buffalo mozzarella
1 tablespoon black olives, chopped
1 tablespoon artichoke heart, chopped
1 cup extra virgin olive oil
1 tablespoon balsamic vinegar

Directions: Marinate chicken overnight in Caesar dressing. Grill chicken, onion, and pepper on stove top or outdoor grill until done. Cut the three grilled ingredients into strips and put in mixing bowl. Add all other ingredients from garlic to artichoke hearts. Toss with 1 cup olive oil and 1 tablespoon balsamic vinegar. Serve chilled with tomato wedges and pita bread or sea salt bagel chips. Makes 6 to 8 servings.

Vegetables pair exceptionally well with herbs. Consult cookbooks for ideal combinations if you are unsure of how to marry flavors and want to get away from simply adding butter. Try this recipe for a tasty way to maximize the flavor of asparagus.

Roasted Asparagus

3   tablespoons olive oil
2   tablespoons balsamic vinegar
1   tablespoon teriyaki sauce
1   tablespoon dried basil
½   teaspoon salt

½   teaspoon black pepper

¼   teaspoon dry mustard

¼   teaspoon nutmeg

1½ pounds fresh asparagus, woody sections trimmed

Directions: Stir together the first eight ingredients in an 11 × 7-inch baking dish. Add asparagus and toss it about to coat. (Use only medium to large stalks as they are more flavorful and better for roasting than thin stalks, which will shrivel up.) Bake covered with foil at 350 degrees F. for 20 minutes, turning asparagus once. Remove with a slotted spoon and serve. Makes 6 to 8 servings.

Hot Stuff!
Herbs for Spicy Cuisine

⇜ by Elizabeth Barrette ⇝

C ertain herbs create a sensation of heat, from a mild tingle to a convincing illusion that you have just set your tongue on fire. In my household, we call such things "food that commands respect." Spanish cleverly distinguishes between the "heat" of ovens (*caliente*) and of spices (*picante*). In recipes, such ingredients add flavorful fireworks. However, different herbs create different flavors and levels of heat. They are used for both savory and sweet dishes. For best results when cooking with picante herbs, you should understand their individual traits.

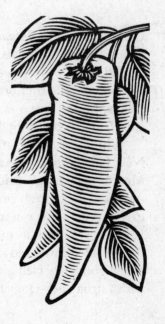

Cinnamon

Cinnamon (*Cinnamomum zeylanicum*) comes from the inner bark of the cinnamon tree, so chances are you can't grow your own. The tree is native to the island of Sri Lanka (formerly Ceylon) and parts of India and Burma. The spice became popular in Europe in the sixteenth century, and has since become widely available.

Cinnamon sticks are the basic form: long curls of bark useful for stirring hot drinks. Powdered cinnamon has a mild to moderate flavor, but becomes bitter if cooked too long. Cinnamon extract and oil are quite powerful—strong enough to burn if spilled on your skin. The flavor of cinnamon comes from a complex blend of phenylpropanoids and other biochemicals.

This spice appears in many spicy-sweet recipes, especially with fruit. It combines well with other warm spices such as allspice, clove, and nutmeg. In small amounts, it merely tastes spicy and sweet. In large amounts, it delivers a respectable nip. I particularly like Saigon cinnamon, a dark-red powder with a strong "redhot" flavor that holds its zing after baking. Also, cinnamon-flavored candies such as Redhots make an excellent ingredient in pies, cookies, stuffed fruits, and other baked goods.

Ginger

Ginger (*Zingiber officinalis*) root is actually a rhizome, or underground stem. It forms plump, knotty sections. Try to find smooth roots with large sections, because they have to be peeled before use. The thin brown skin comes away to reveal a bright yellow, fibrous interior. When preparing fresh ginger, remove any "hairs" you may find.

This herb originated in the East Indies, Malaysia, and New Guinea before gradually spreading throughout Asia, the Mediterranean and Middle East, the Caribbean, and parts of America. Today, fresh ginger root is readily available and relatively easy to grow—you can sprout roots bought at a grocery store.

Ginger comes in many forms, and they're not very interchangeable. Powdered ginger is mild, good in spice blends and baked goods. Pickled ginger comes in bright pink, floppy slices with a strong hot-tangy flavor—an ideal condiment for sushi and other dishes. Candied ginger is intensely hot and sweet; I like to eat it right out of the bag, but most people chop it fine and add it to cookies or ice cream. Fresh ginger root (usually sliced, chopped, or grated) and fresh ginger juice are the hottest—a pure golden fire. Don't prepare fresh ginger and then rub your eyes! It works equally well with fresh fruits or vegetables, and for cooking. Ginger beer (which is alcohol free) ranges from mild to vehement and makes an excellent base for beverages, dressings, and marinades. Good ginger beer leaves a pleasant tingle on your tongue and a warmth in your mouth; great ginger beer atomizes your gullet on the way down. Jamaican brands are usually the strongest. For the most ginger flavor in a recipe, combine two or more forms of the herb.

Pear-Ginger Ice Cream

3   fresh pears
1   tablespoon lemon juice
3   inches fresh ginger root
⅔   cup sugar
1   cup whole milk
1   cup heavy cream

Choose soft, juicy pears. Peel and coarsely chop them, then put the pieces in a blender. Add the lemon juice. Peel the ginger root and slice it thinly, then add it to the blender. Pulse to liquefy. Pour into large bowl. Add sugar and stir until it dissolves. Stir in the milk and heavy cream. Pour into ice cream machine and freeze about 30 minutes. This ice cream has a sweet, creamy flavor with sparkly notes from the ginger. Makes about 1 quart.

Horseradish

Horseradish (*Cochlearia amoracia*) belongs to the cabbage family. Its long, slender roots are nearly cylindrical with patches of tiny "hairs." The thin outer skin is pale yellow; the interior is almost white and intensely pungent. Roots must be washed and peeled before use, then they may be grated or sliced thinly.

Originally from southeastern Europe, horseradish now flourishes throughout much of Europe and North America. It grows easily in most gardens. This herb appears in historic records from Egyptian, Greek, and Hebrew cultures. Its culinary and medicinal use dates back at least as far as 1500 BC.

Horseradish delivers the greatest strength when used fresh and raw. It combines well with heavy cream, sour cream, cream cheese, or butter to make a variety of smooth, sharp sauces. Dried, powdered horseradish has some zing and is easy to store. Commercial "horseradish sauce" typically blends the root with vinegar, oil, and other spices. The sauce loses potency over time. Cooking also weakens the impact of horseradish considerably.

Mustard

Mustard seeds come from the *Cruciferae* family and there are three main kinds: black (strongest, but rare), brown (moderate and uncommon), and yellow (mild and common). Black mustard is from Asia and the Middle East; brown mustard is Asian; yellow mustard is Mediterranean. Mustard has been used in much of Europe for centuries, and its cultivation has spread to America.

Sometimes you can find actual mustard seeds. Mostly, your choices will be mustard powder or commercial mustard sauce made with vinegar, water, and other spices. The active components in mustard seeds that give mustard its pungent flavor are glucoside and the enzyme myrosin, which are released when the seeds are crushed and mixed with water. However, boiling water turns myrosin bitter, so use cold water for mustard.

Mustard also loses some of its flavor with long cooking and high heat, so it's best when added near the end of the cooking time. It makes a fine sauce, and commercial mustard sauce is a good thickener. Honey mustard is mostly sugar, so it carmelizes when heated—ideal for putting a sweet-hot brown coating on meat and poultry.

Onions

Onions (*Allium cepa*) probably originated in Central or West Asia. They have been used in Europe since the Bronze Age. Onions are easy to grow and now appear in much of the world. They store very well, and have long been an important winter food.

Onions come in various colors and flavors. Red onions tend to be the mildest, with a peppery-sweet taste; they add color to salads and salsas. White onions are hotter, and some yellow ones are downright sharp. These are good for cooking. However, yellow Vidalia onions are quite mild and sweet, excellent raw on salads or sandwiches. All onions lose much of their heat when cooked, but retain an "oniony" flavor. They are often sautéed in butter or oil and then added to recipes.

Fresh onions are by far the hottest form and are best for most uses. Dried minced onion is easy to store, however, and acceptable in stews or other cooked foods if you want onion flavor more than heat. Onion salt or onion powder may also give some flavor. The active components of onion, which make your eyes water when you cut one, include sulfur compounds and flavonoides. These also give onions their characteristic "stinky" smell.

Peppercorns

The pepper vine (*Piper nigrum*) yields several colors of peppercorns depending on preparation. Classic black peppercorns are picked just before they start to redden, then sun-dried. Green peppercorns are picked while still unripe, then dried or pickled. White peppercorns are picked ripe, then soaked to remove the blackened skin, and finally dried. Black pepper tends to be hottest. Green pepper has a lively taste that nicely complements delicate flavors. White pepper is milder, and ideal when black specks would look unappetizing. Fresh-ground pepper is always zestier than preground powder.

Red peppercorns are different. They primarily come from a South American tree often known as the Brazilian peppertree

(*Schinus terebinthifolius*). Picked when nearly ripe, these dry to a pink or red color. They are more aromatic and complex than black peppercorns, mildly hot, with a fruity flavor that goes very well in sweet dishes that just need a little zip.

The pepper vine is native to India, but peppercorns quickly became popular (and expensive) in Europe. Pepper was a vital part of the spice trade and helped fuel the demand for a shorter and faster route between Europe and India. Today pepper grows in India, Cambodia, Brazil, Madagascar, and several other places.

Interestingly, the texture of peppercorns affects their use in foods. Fine pepper powder has a subtle flavor and is used in delicate dishes. Medium-ground pepper is used most often and it works in most recipes. Coarse-ground pepper is best on salads and soups—most tabletop pepper grinders are coarse. It's also used in "blackened" or "peppered" recipes for coating meats. Whole peppercorns can go into pickling brine, stocks, and stews.

Peppers

Peppers belong to the *Capsicum* genus. There are hundreds of varieties, from mild bell peppers to incendiary habañeros. A special scale has been invented to define how hot certain peppers are: Scoville Heat Units. This refers to how much water is required to dilute a sample of the pepper before the taste vanishes.

The pepper species originated in Central and South America, with some varieties in the West Indies also. Peppers had been used by Aztecs, Mayans, and Indians for centuries before the Spanish discovered them in the 1400s. Peppers thrived in the Mediterranean climate. They have since spread over much of America and Europe, Africa, India, and the Far East; but the plants still grow best in hot, dry habitats.

Most peppers are hotter when fresh. However, some intensify with drying. Small, narrow peppers with pointed ends tend to be hotter than larger, broader ones. The active component is capcaicin oil, which is very persistent if you get it on your hands. It can burn skin or mucous membranes at high concentrations. It breaks down somewhat with long cooking, but overall, most pepper flavor stands up just fine when heated. Most of the capcaicin concentrates in the ribs and seeds of a pepper, rather than the flesh, so removing those can lessen the heat.

Some peppers have particular uses. Jalapeños are often cooked and stuffed, or sliced and pickled. Serranos and chilies are excellent dried, and store well in that form. Mild bell peppers may be used fresh in salads, or cooked and stuffed. Habañeros are wickedly hot, either fresh or dried; a tiny fraction will replace a much larger amount of crushed red peppers. Another devastating fireball is the minute chile pequin, which grows wild along the Mexican border, and often finds its way into chili recipes. For the most part, though, any pepper whose flavor you like can be swapped into most pepper recipes.

Dragon Eggs

15	large, fresh jalapeños
4	ounces cream cheese
2	tablespoons lemon juice
1	teaspoon onion salt
1	small can chopped meat (ham, tuna, chicken, etc.)
½	cup shredded sharp cheddar cheese

Split peppers lengthwise on one side. Carefully remove seeds and ribs, leaving stem attached. Rinse peppers, drain, and allow to dry for an hour. Beat cream cheese until fluffy. Mix in lemon juice and onion salt. Mix in chopped meat. Using a spoon, fill each pepper with cream cheese mixture. Arrange on baking sheet. Top the split side of peppers with the shredded cheddar. Bake at 350 degrees F. for 8 to 10 minutes or until cheese melts. Serves 15.

Radishes

Radishes (*Raphanus sativus*) probably evolved from the wild radish (*Raphanus raphanistrum*), a native of Europe and a common weed worldwide. It was domesticated in the eastern Mediterranean area prior to 2780 BC. Growing in various shapes and colors, most radish roots are either spherical or long and tapering. Colors include shades of red, pink, white, and black. The thin, smooth skin may be scrubbed clean and left intact, or peeled off.

These roots are usually eaten fresh, although Asian recipes sometimes cook them. They add a sharp, peppery flavor and a crunchy, slightly juicy texture. Use them in salads, stir-fries, and other dishes made with fresh herbs and vegetables.

Healing Properties

Picante herbs and spices share some general properties relating to health. They tend to be germicidal; the active components in hot foods are pretty aggressive. The "heat" causes your sinuses to drain and may also cause sweating, which can be good for colds.

Spicy foods also share a warming, invigorating effect. Eat them in autumn and winter to stoke your inner fires, both physically and emotionally.

Cinnamon is an antimicrobial that also improves digestive health and helps balance blood sugar. The invigorating scent boosts brain function.

Ginger aids digestion and soothes upset stomachs. It also stimulates circulation and clears congestion in the lungs.

Horseradish is a strong antimicrobial often used in picnic foods to slow the growth of organisms that cause food poisoning.

Mustard is anti-inflammatory, so it may reduce the symptoms of arthritis and gout. The seeds also provide numerous vitamins and nutrients.

Onions can improve cardiovascular and gastrointestinal health. They are anti-inflammatory and anti-bacterial.

Peppercorns aid digestion by stimulating stomach secretions and reducing gas. They also contain antioxidants.

Peppers help fight colds and bronchial infections.

Radishes are high in vitamin C, which helps prevent asthma attacks and makes the skin less susceptible to bruising.

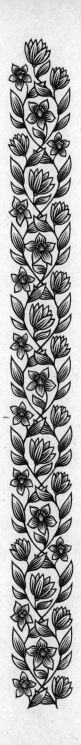

Herbs
for
Health

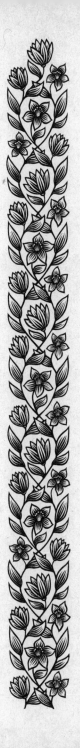

The Happy Traveler

≫ by Chandra Moira Beal ≪

Travel is a wonderful way to expand your horizons. Exploring the planet allows you to experience other cultures, sample new cuisines, and gain a greater perspective. Whether for pleasure or work—or both—traveling can be exciting and adventurous.

But travel can have a stressful side, too. Changing time zones, sitting for long periods, and navigating foreign situations can leave you feeling vulnerable to illness. But with a little preparation and using nature's resources, you can ensure a great experience.

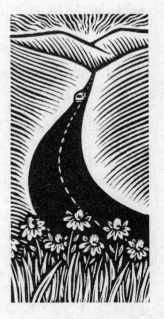

Before You Go

A successful trip begins before you walk out the door. Take some time to prepare your body for the journey by strengthening your immune and digestive systems. A few days before departure, take ligustrum and astragalus, which are excellent tonic herbs. Ligustrum berries help to boost energy and are effective when heat and fatigue combine to make you feel worn down. They nourish the liver and kidneys and help perk you up. Astragalus root is a powerful but gentle tonic that fortifies the immune system while strengthening digestion and raising metabolism. Paired together, these two herbs make a potent immune booster and restorative.

If it's cold and flu season, echinacea and thyme should be your traveling companions. Echinacea, a well-known immune defender and stimulator, increases the body's disease-fighting components that provide a barrier against illness. Besides increasing the supply of white blood cells to an infected area, echinacea is also antibiotic and antibacterial, fighting against streptococcus or staphylococcus. Thyme is an antiseptic plant that is useful for fighting fungal, bacterial, and viral illnesses. Place a couple of drops of thyme essential oil in four ounces of water as a mouthwash for a toothache or sore throat. Two drops placed in steaming water can be inhaled for colds, flu, or bronchitis.

Watch Your Diet

Travel often means disrupted routines and eating habits. We tend to eat richer foods and larger meals, or foods prepared without Western sanitation standards. By toning up your digestive system and gut you'll be less vulnerable to gastric upsets and more able to enjoy local cuisine, such as street-vendor meals. When dining out, choose dishes that make use of culinary herbs like ginger, garlic, and onions, all of which are all immune-strengthening as well as tasty.

Artichoke leaves are a good choice for the digestive system as they increase the production of bile, which assists in digesting fats via the liver and gallbladder. Gentian stimulates the production of saliva and gastric juices, which helps break down and assimilate nutrients. Gentian also helps balance the pancreas, which helps us regulate blood-sugar levels and maintain a healthy appetite.

Aloe vera is excellent for the gut and stomach flora and reduces inflammation in the body. Take aloe vera concentrate made from the inner part of the leaf—the most potent part of the plant.

Getting There

For most of us, adventures begin with boarding a plane, train, automobile, or boat, yet for some this can be the least pleasant part of the trip. Motion sickness, nausea, and jet lag can leave you feeling like curling up in bed instead of heading out to see the sights.

To ease stomach upsets and nausea, ginger is a great all-around herb that is readily available in supermarkets. The juices in the root soothe upset stomachs and cramps, and have warming qualities that stimulate circulation. Ginger is most effective when fresh, so make some ginger tea before you leave and fill a Thermos to take with you. Use one grated tablespoon of the root for every eight ounces of boiling water, letting it steep for five minutes. If you are traveling by air and can't take liquids in the cabin, you can also take ginger freeze-dried in capsules, or as an extract that you can mix into water after you board. Pack a few ginger tea bags in your carry on and ask for hot water during the beverage service. Peppermint and fennel teas are also soothing for the tummy, so pack a few extra tea bags containing these herbs.

If your upset stomach is accompanied by vomiting or diarrhea, then a blend of goldenseal tincture and chamomile tincture can be a lifesaver. These herbs not only tackle infection but also help repair and soothe the stomach lining. Your symptoms may continue even after taking this formula because the goldenseal keeps working until all bacteria in the gut and stomach are ejected. Chamomile then settles the stomach. Slippery elm is another useful herb for upset stomachs. If you suspect food poisoning, capsules of slippery elm powder combine and buffer poisons in the stomach and bowels to decrease toxic absorption. It can soothe mucous membranes and settle a cramped stomach. Be sure to increase your water intake if you have stomach upset while traveling to avoid dehydration.

If your symptoms persist and you suspect you've picked up a parasite, artemisia is capable of disarming a wide range of pathological microorganisms. While not a cure, artemisia can be an excellent support measure until a doctor can see you.

During a long flight, the body is especially vulnerable to dehydration, while also being exposed to oxygen imbalances, radiation, reduced circulation, and sleep disturbances. The immune system is further burdened by the close proximity to other people who may be unwell. All these elements can contribute to the feelings of tiredness, stress, and general imbalance that we call jet lag.

Jet lag can be reduced by using Siberian ginseng tincture. Ginseng is an adaptogenic herb, which means it balances all the organs and systems within the body and has a diverse and positive effect. Siberian ginseng is a fantastic tonic for the adrenals and an immune booster, stimulating resistance to mental and physical stress. Ginseng can help normalize blood-sugar levels, and protect against radiation while flying. Siberian ginseng was even used in the aftermath of the Chernobyl disaster in the 1980s to help protect against radiation damage.

Peppermint is another friend to take along during a long flight. A few drops of the essential oil rubbed into the temples can help you stay awake so you can regulate your sleep cycle on arrival, and taking a few drops with water will settle an upset stomach.

If you find you retain water after a long flight, consider taking dandelion or marshmallow extracts (or parsley and cornsilk herbal tea). These herbs are all diuretics which will help balance fluid levels.

Outdoor Fun

When you finally reach your destination, it's easy to plunge headlong into hours of sightseeing, hiking, or just lounging by the pool. But you should continue to care for your body so you can enjoy your trip to the very last day.

Protecting your skin from overexposure to the sun is common sense these days. Don't ruin your vacation on the first day by getting sunburned! Sun protection also helps prevent premature aging and skin problems associated with exposure to sun, like blotching and pigmentation imbalances.

There are several brands of natural, paraben-, and PABA-free sunscreens on the market now. Cocoa butter and sesame oil are considered natural sunscreens and will nourish your skin at the same time. Wear a hat and try to stay out of the sun between 10 am and 4 pm, which is when the rays are the strongest.

If you do get burned, aloe vera gel is excellent for soothing and naturally restoring the skin. Lavender essential oil can be applied directly to burned skin for relief, too. Comfrey, calendula, and plantain are also soothing herbs for the skin. Plantain leaves gathered wild can be crushed and the juice applied directly to the skin. And don't forget to protect your lips. Fresh aloe vera can be smoothed onto the lips to relieve dryness and cracking.

Insects are absolutely essential to the balance of life on this planet, but they can be downright annoying. Before your trip, mix your own insect repellent in a spray bottle containing distilled water and rubbing alcohol. Add several drops of the essential oils of lavender, citronella, eucalyptus, cedar wood, and lemongrass. This combination is pleasant smelling to humans, but noxious to bugs. Combining these herbs works better than the single oils on their own. (Note that many herbal insect repellents suggest pennyroyal, but this herb has proven dangerous to pregnant women and pets.)

Perhaps your holiday involves strenuous exercise, such as hiking or skiing. Maybe you spend all day walking through city streets taking in the sights. Either way, you are bound to have tired legs and feet at the end of the day. Arnica is an excellent herb for relieving muscle aches and pains, and can be taken internally in homeopathically prepared pellets or applied topically as a gel or lotion. Do not use arnica on broken skin.

You can also make a liniment for external use with arnica, witch hazel, and St. John's wort tinctures with essential oils of camphor, eucalyptus, rosemary, and clove bud. This makes a nice warming rub for tired and sore muscles.

If you've developed blisters from walking, aloe vera gel and lavender essential oil applied to the surface will help them heal.

Wherever you go and whatever you do, remember to call on nature's bounty to enrich your experience and make your journeys enjoyable.

The Herbal First-Aid Kit

Take some time to build a simple herbal first-aid kit using just a few basic ingredients. The contents are versatile and will prove useful around the house. Having these items at hand can be indispensable while you're traveling.

Lavender Essential Oil

Lavender is the only essential oil you can put directly on a minor burn. Immediately run the affected area under cold water for as long as possible, then dab some lavender oil over the burn. Lavender is also good for healing bruises, reducing swelling around sprains, and soothing on cuts and insect bites. Lavender helps with emotional and mental stress, too. Apply a few drops to the temples and wrists if you are feeling stressed or unsettled.

Aloe Vera Gel

Taking fresh aloe vera leaves with you on a trip or keeping them in a first-aid kit may be impractical, so invest in some fresh, pure "inner leaf" gel in a bottle. This will keep well and can be used to soothe and heal minor burns, sunburns, and blisters. Taken internally, aloe vera gel can help repair stomach lining after an illness.

Arnica

Include both homeopathic arnica for internal use, and an arnica gel or lotion in your first-aid kit. The gel makes a great massage liniment for sore and cramped muscles. It will decrease pain and prevent swelling and bruising associated with torn ligaments, sprains, crushed fingers and toes, and broken bones. Arnica works best if applied immediately after an injury and reapplied every couple of hours for the first day. The internal pellets are useful for reducing muscle soreness from sitting too long or overexerting oneself, such as when carrying heavy bags.

Tea Tree Essential Oil

Favored by Australians for its antibacterial and antiseptic properties, tea tree oil is a must-have in your herbal first-aid kit. It will be astringent on a wound, but very effective for keeping it clean, particularly if you want to cover it with a bandage. Never apply tea tree oil directly onto broken skin—dilute it in a little water, soak a cotton ball in the solution, and dab that on the wound.

Thyme Essential Oil

Thyme is essential for camping trips when you are likely to encounter bugs. Place two drops in four ounces of water and use externally for crabs, lice, and all external parasites. Two drops placed in recently boiled water can be inhaled to relieve symptoms of cold, flu, or bronchitis.

Echinacea Extract

If you feel yourself coming down with cold or flu symptoms, reach for echinacea extract to boost your immune system. Take it in a tea, glass of water, or apply a few drops under the tongue.

Siberian Ginseng Extract

Helpful with jet lag symptoms or when you need a boost, such as during a long drive, Siberian ginseng extract can be taken in water, juice, or tea.

Ginger

Place a few freeze-dried ginger capsules or dried ginger tea bags in your emergency kit for upset stomachs, gas, or nausea.

Tea Bags

Place a few herbal tea bags each of peppermint leaf, fennel, ginger, and chamomile tea inside a sealed plastic bag. These are all yummy tasting herbs that will soothe upset stomachs, aid digestion, help calm nerves, and ensure good sleep.

Antimicrobial Healing Salve

This is something you'll want to make ahead of time to have on hand. Heat about two ounces of oil (olive, almond, or coconut are good choices). Grate two tablespoons of beeswax into the pan. Add a pinch each of powdered comfrey, plantain, St. John's wort, calendula, and echinacea, plus a few drops each of lavender and rosemary oils. Mix together and let it cool, then store in a lidded jar. This is a good, all-purpose salve which will decrease swelling and fight bacteria as well as soothe, accelerate healing, and disinfect any cuts, scratches, and burns.

Pain Relievers

Meadowsweet tincture and white willow bark are known to be fast acting, anti-inflammatory painkillers. Also bring a few aspirin.

Valerian Tincture

As an antispasmodic and painkiller, this herb relieves intestinal and menstrual cramps, headaches, and general aches or pains. As a nervine, it will bring sleep to an exhausted person.

Hardware

In addition to your herbal arsenal, throw in a few bandages, cotton balls, small scissors, tweezers, an Ace bandage, and an instant cold pack. Pack it inside a waterproof case, and you've got yourself a great herbal first-aid kit!

Herbs for Young Children

✺ by Clea Danaan ✺

After I squirted the dark, mysterious-looking liquid into my toddler's mouth, she tasted it, and promptly signed, "More." Chocolate? Molasses? Nope. This coveted potion was in fact cough medicine, made by mama in the kitchen with herbs. The vegetable glycerin base had masked all the bitterness of the elecampane and muted the spicy ginger root, resulting in a sweet syrup that my baby was happy to swallow. I felt like Mary Poppins, pouring a spoonful of magical-flavored medicine to ease the normal but not-so-fun challenges of childhood.

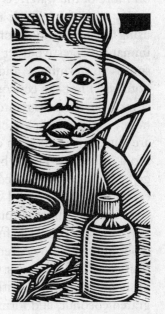

Making your own herbal-based children's medicines is easy as tea and cake. With simple ingredients found at your local health-food store, you can mix up candies, Popsicles, and teas to support your child's immune system, ease restless sleep, soothe teething's painful bite, and more. The few times I have used a conventional over-the-counter children's medicine, I have felt accosted by the too-sticky smell, fake flavors, and high-fructose-corn syrup. While I do use conventional medicines at times, I realize they are usually only suppressing symptoms, not supporting the body to heal itself. This is why most of the time, I prefer herbal remedies.

I find the easiest way to administer herbal remedies is syrup, with either a baby medicine dropper or a spoon. To make your own syrup, first decoct the herbs of choice (recipes to follow) by simmering in water over gentle heat for twenty minutes or so. Strain the mixture, tossing the herbs into the compost, then return the resulting thick tea to the stove. Stir in half as much honey or vegetable glycerin, and let thicken a little over low heat. Cooking very long can kill off some of the beneficial enzymes in honey, so I just let it simmer a short time to blend and evaporate off more of the water. As a general rule, I use vegetable glycerin in any syrup for infants; after one year of age, I feel comfortable using honey. (Honey contains spores that a very young baby's immature digestive tract cannot fully break down, allowing the spores to germinate and release toxins that can cause infant botulism.) Let the concoction cool and pour into a jar. You can store it in the refrigerator for six weeks, possibly more. Since honey and glycerin are both preservatives, the chances of mold are slim, but it's best to check your remedies regularly for any mold or mildew just to be safe. However, I have never had one go bad before we finished it, even when we kept it in the refrigerator for an entire cold season.

Candy is another fun way to administer herbal medicines. This works best with fully powdered herbs. Combine a few tablespoons of powdered herbal mixture with nuts and dried fruits in a food processor until a gummy, figlike substance forms. Or mix herb powders with nut butter and honey, blend in a little grated coconut, and form into balls. Roll in powdered cocoa or carob, and enjoy! I also store these in the refrigerator, but since all ingredients are fine at room temperature, they will last for months before going stale even sitting on the counter.

Pleasant-tasting herbs like lemon balm can be made into tea for children, administered in a bottle or sippy cup when cooled. The tea can also be frozen into herbal popsicles, a favorite for young children and teething toddlers. Root herbs, like ginger or dandelion root, need to be decocted longer in gently simmering water, while leaves and flowers can steep in a covered cup of hot water just like tea. Herbal teas should steep longer than your morning cup of Earl Grey to extract all the active constituents. For children's remedies, the tea can be made fairly bland by using fewer herbs than you would for yourself. Blend in a little honey or stevia if you like, then drink warm or freeze in popsicle molds.

If an adult dosage of herbs would be one cup, give a child younger than two years a teaspoon or less. Increase to two teaspoons for a child between two and four years of age; four to seven-years gets one tablespoon; and at seven to eleven years old, administer two tablespoons. If the adult dosage is a teaspoon, as with a syrup, start with only two drops of syrup for younger than three months, and increase by a drop every three months. At two years of age, a child can take ten drops, increasing by two to three drops each year. Popsicles can be made to taste, since you will be using very gentle herbs like catnip and lemon balm, which are safe at larger doses.

Recipes

Here are a few recipes for the herbal remedies I have used with my toddler. I am not terribly strict about my measuring and tend to just grab a bunch of this and a pinch of that, then cover with water. So feel free to adjust to your tastes and needs.

Cough and Cold Syrup

Blend a couple of tablespoons of dried licorice root with a tablespoon each of cinnamon, echinacea, elecampane, and a pinch of ginger. Add optional tablespoons of lemon balm, rose hips, elderberries, or clover flowers for additional respiratory and immune support. Elecampane and elderberries are the two herbs I turn to specifically for respiratory and cold support; the others help ease cold, flu, and cough symptoms while nourishing the whole body. For a simpler cold remedy, just make an elderberry and echinacea blend.

Pour three cups of water over these herbs, enough to cover them plus extra water that will evaporate. Simmer on low heat for at least twenty minutes, and follow the above directions for making a syrup. Administer appropriate dosages for the age of your child several times a day.

Calcium Tea

Babies grow extremely fast, adding bone mass and teeth daily. Extra calcium can help support strong bones and teeth, and helps reduce growing pains and muscle spasms. A tasty high-calcium tea can be made from tablespoon-sized pinches of rose hips, lemon balm, lemongrass, oats (actual oats or oat straw), nettle, and raspberry leaf. Flavor with cinnamon and honey or stevia. Serve as a room temperature tea or freeze in a popsicle.

Thrush Remedy

My daughter contracted a nasty sore throat, and we decided the best course of action was to give her antibiotics. The illness cleared up, but a few weeks later she developed thrush. The antibiotics had caused an imbalance of flora in her system, and she got thrushy white fungus in her mouth and a terrible diaper rash. To heal the Candida growth, I swiped her mouth several times a day with yogurt, powdered probiotics made for children, and baking soda (one at a time, not all at once). I soothed her diaper rash with lavender and tea tree essential oils. I also fed her lots of breast milk and gave her a few drops of echinacea tea daily. The thrush cleared up completely within a week, and has not returned.

Bum Salve

One of the first herbal remedies I made my daughter was bum salve, which I whipped up while she still turned in my belly. Over low heat I infused a few tablespoons of olive oil with calendula and lavender, which are soothing and antiseptic. I then strained the herbal oil, and put it back on the stove with a few tablespoons of beeswax. When the beeswax melted completely into the oil, I poured the mixture into little salve jars, and set them on the changing table to await my daughter's birth. She was not the only one who used this healing salve, however, as my husband and I also found it useful for chapped lips, rashes, and hangnails.

Colic and Sleeplessness Therapies

My sweet babe had a gentle birth, was worn in a sling regularly, and slept with us. Despite this loving entry, she had a few difficulties transitioning from the spirit world. Her distress showed up as lots of crying and frequent night waking. Besides walking in circles while bouncing our baby at all hours of the day and night, we found a few herbal remedies helpful during this challenging time.

A few drops of gripe water helped soothe her undeveloped digestive system. Gripe water is usually a little fennel and ginger in vegetable glycerin, though there are several recipes to choose from. Simple fennel tea can also help. Give baby a few drops from a medicine dropper.

Lemon balm, catnip, and chamomile are nervine tonics, easing the brand-new, very sensitive nervous system. These herbs can be useful throughout childhood during times of transition and stress (which is most of childhood, really). Lemon balm is the top herb for use in children, as it is a nervine, antimicrobial, and carminative, meaning it helps calm gas. Catnip soothes and sedates, reduces pain, lowers fevers, and aids digestion. It is a little bitter, so is best combined with lemon balm, rose, and chamomile. Chamomile is anti-inflammatory, and calms the nervous and digestive systems while toning the immune system.

The breastfeeding mother can also take these calming herbs herself in stronger teas and add hops and valerian. Listening to a screaming baby and waking up every two hours at night wears on a mother's nervous system. These herbs will help calm you, and your baby will get small doses of the herbs through your milk.

Childhood Health Tactics

My all-time favorite herbal for childhood remedies is Rosemary Gladstar's *Family Herbal: A Guide to Living Life with Energy, Health, and Vitality*. I turn to her at the first sign of distress in any of my family members. But sometimes herbs and mama love are not enough, and I need to call my pediatrician. How do you know when you need professional help? If your child seems to be losing steam under the pressure of the invading illness, if her eyes are cloudy and she has little energy, then go get help. I sometimes find among natural-minded parents a feeling of failure if you go to a doctor—especially if you administer antibiotics or other strong medication. There are so many things to feel guilty about—caring for your child appropriately is not one of them. Use herbs to support, nourish, and ease; and when you need it, which you likely will at some point, your doctor's knowledge is invaluable. Antibiotics and other medications are not wrong, just to be used when appropriate. Furthermore, if your child has any special conditions, like allergies, autism, or serious sleep disturbances, work with a knowledgeable, herb-friendly doctor to determine the most effective and safe herbal remedies.

Nourishing your child with gentle herbal remedies will give her two invaluable gifts. First, you strengthen and support the body, giving it tools to heal itself. With future illnesses, then, the immune and nervous systems can retain balance more easily and quickly. Second, you teach your child about the power and sacredness of plants, and about her connection to the Earth. With a simple berry syrup, you not only heal a child, but the Earth as well. Pretty powerful mama magic!

Bolstering Breastfeeding

～ by Clea Danaan ～

I pushed open the door to the shop and stepped out of the chilly wind. A little bell jingled, welcoming me to the herb-scented sanctuary. Handmade antique pedestals sported baggies of salt scrubs and nourishing teas. Fairies danced on a twig display on the front counter, and tiny white lights twinkled along the walls. I let a little of my chronic tension go like drips of dew into a river.

It was my first night out alone without my new baby. I had left her with her papa, and made the trek across town to MoonDance Botanicals for a spa party with four other mamas. The store owner, herbalist Tonja Reichley, guided us through a scrumptious array of handmade soaps, cleansers, and herbal treatments for our faces.

Spending time just with myself and other women, wrapped in the spicy,

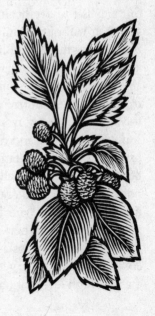

soothing embrace of herbs felt like a homecoming. When we got the facial steam, I covered my head with a line-dried, wind-scented towel, and allowed the herby steam to purify my pores. The last of the new-mama tension I had carried into the store evaporated with the steam, and I almost began to cry. It was as if through the message of these sweet-scented herbs and the fire of the purified steam, a goddess had laid a hand on my shoulder and assured me all would be all right. I would survive the spiritual initiation of motherhood, from the sleepless nights to round-the-clock nursing and the search for my own private self in the midst of a new identity.

Since that night, I have tried to give myself regular herbal facials and renewed my dedication to drinking nourishing herbal teas. The shining green power of herbs has helped me immensely in this intense time of new motherhood.

Nutrition and Nursing

Herbs are especially useful for nursing mothers. A lactating mom gives her child optimum nutrition, energy, and emotional support. She needs to have healthy reserves of all three in order to give so much without burning out. Here is one area our little green friends, the herbs, can help. Herbs can nourish the body, mind, and spirit of the new mama while she in turn nurtures her babe.

Human milk is something of a miracle substance, drawing from a mother's nutrients to provide exactly the right nutrition for a growing baby from birth through weaning. The immune support, minerals, and vitamins a child receives from human milk provide a solid foundation that will stay with the growing child beyond weaning as well. Even poor nutrition in a mother does not lead to poor milk, but actually to a malnourished mother. To help ourselves and our babies, and to supplement the foods we eat, we can turn to herbs.

My favorite herbs as a breastfeeding mother include nettle, comfrey, red raspberry leaf, and clover. These herbs are relaxing, contain high levels of nutrients like calcium, folic acid, and iron.

And they taste good. Nettle supports the whole body, strengthens the blood, and is high in iron, vitamin C, and chlorophyll. It tastes good as a hot or iced tea, and can be cooked in stir-fries, casseroles, and omelets. Combine a tablespoon of nettle with a tablespoon of comfrey, clover, or raspberry leaf, or any combination of the above herbs. Place two tablespoons or more of this mixture in a cup, cover with at least eight ounces of boiling water, and steep for fifteen minutes for a nurturing mama tea.

Calcium Tea

A milk-making mama needs extra calcium to replace what is given to her child. Rosemary Gladstar offers a tasty calcium tea in *Family Herbal*. This can be given to teething or growing children as well as the nursing mother.

3   parts rose hips

2   parts lemon balm

2   parts lemon grass

2   parts oats

1   part nettle

1   part raspberry leaf

½   part cinnamon

Pinch of stevia to sweeten (optional)

Combine herbs and store in an airtight container. To make the tea, put a tablespoon or so per cup of water in a tea basket, and cover with boiling water. Cover water, steep for about 15 minutes, and enjoy.

Milk Production

To increase milk flow, try fennel, borage, blessed thistle, and hops. These can be made into a tea, or taken as a tincture. Find prepared tinctures specifically for the nursing mother at health food stores, or make your own by mixing a tablespoon or two of each herb together and covering with vodka or vegetable glycerin until the liquid rises a few inches above the surface of the herbs. Keep in an airtight jar for six weeks, shaking the mixture daily. Infuse the tincture with positive thoughts of mother love. Strain the mixture after six weeks, store in a dark glass jar, and take a dropper full daily in a glass of water.

Energy and Emotion

I hold my nursling in my arms, in front of my heart. The sound of my breath and heartbeat, the rhythm of sucking, and our perfectly focused gaze wrap us both in a soothing embrace. Energy flows from my heart, my hands, and my crown chakra into this tiny person as she nurses.

And then when she finishes, she climbs out of my lap and runs across the room, laughing. She does a somersault and calls, "Up!" I lift her twenty pounds and go about our day.

From the calm moments to the hyper fun, I exert more energy as a mother than I ever have before. I support her until I am exhausted, and then keep holding her, playing with her, and giving her nourishing milk. At the end of the day, my own nervous system needs some support. My favorite herbs for calming the nerves and opening the heart include lavender, lemon balm, rosemary, and skullcap.

Lavender helps alleviate headaches and mild depression. It calms stress and eases insomnia. I use a pinch of it in my nettle tea or sprinkle a few drops of the essential oil in the bath—or even right on my temples. The smell itself can make me happy.

Lemon balm tastes lovely in tea, sorbet, and cooked in rice. It is antispasmodic, antiviral, and calming. It can be used as a mild sedative, easing the exhausted body and helping us sleep.

Rosemary reduces high blood pressure and tones the nervous system. It soothes the skin and aids circulation. Use it in cooking or include a pinch in your tea. Include a drop or two of rosemary essential oil in your bathwater to cleanse and protect.

Skullcap is my favorite herb to aid sleep when mixed with valerian. It is a very effective nervine and sedative. It renews and revives the central nervous system and eases exhaustion and depression. It is safe to use in large doses but is somewhat bitter, so is best combined with lavender and lemon balm or a little honey when used in a tea.

Motherwort is another lovely herb for nervous support. Herbalist Tonja Reichley says, "I also love motherwort (*Leonurus cardiaca*) . . . great during any time of transition for a woman, a power herb and its name says it all!" Wort means herb or plant, and this cardiac tonic is antispasmodic and sedative. A lovely wort for a mother. Motherwort is also rather bitter and can be taken in capsules, tinctures, or mixed with tastier herbs in tea. It goes nicely with nettle, raspberry leaf, and a little honey.

Reconnecting with Yourself

Not only does a nursing mother need nutritional and physical support, but a regular time to return to herself. When we become mothers, we say goodbye to the maiden we once were, and forge a new self as a woman. We do not have time, though, for meditation retreats and long quiet walks by the sea to reconnect with our inner self. One way I have found to rediscover stillness and nourish my soul is to take ten minutes to give myself an herbal steam.

Wash your face with a gentle cleanser. To exfoliate, blend almond meal or poppy seeds with honey, a touch of almond oil, and lavender flowers. Honey is a humectant, meaning it helps your skin retain moisture. It also has antimicrobial and antiseptic qualities and can be used as a preservative. Lavender soothes the skin and provides additional antibacterial agents.

Now place a healthy handful of any combination of the following herbs in a bowl, and cover with boiling water. Lean over the bowl, and cover your head with a towel to trap the herbal healing steam around your skin. The steam is hot, so adjust your distance from the water and the closeness of the towel for comfort and safety. Here are some herbs to try:

Rose petals   Comfrey
Calendula   Chamomile
Lavender flowers   Raspberry leaf
Sage   Rosemary

If you use essential oils in your steam, utilize only a drop, because the oils are very strong and can be overpowering.

When I sit in the steamy herb temple under my towel, I feel infused with the earthy power of the herbs and the cleansing light of the sun. I take deep breaths and give thanks for the gift of healing, purification, and transmutation offered by my herbal allies. I feel reconnected with my path as an incarnated soul. When I remove the towel, splash my face with rosewater, and rub a gentle cream into my glowing skin, I feel ready to step back into the most difficult, most important, and most rewarding job of all time, motherhood.

A New Perspective

I started working with herbs as a teenager, but until I became a mother, I did not fully appreciate their power to nurture, strengthen, and heal. Whether taken internally in tinctures or teas, or used in beauty products like scrubs and steams, herbs wrap me in a loving embrace just as I hold my daughter. These green allies carry the light of the sun, the dark of the soil, and the power of the universe to guide and make whole. I highly recommend to any new or expecting mother that you find a good herbal resource (www.kellymom.com and www.moondancebotanicals. com are good places to start) and a trusted herbalist in your area to help you through the greatest transition of your life.

The Untold Story of St. John's Wort

❧ by Cheryl Hoard ❧

An ornament of meadows, St. John's wort is a beautiful, yellow-blooming shrub that doesn't demand much for its survival. It even has a presence at an altitude of ten thousand feet, where many other plants refuse to live. Often found growing comfortably in woods basking in speckled shade and sun, this herb really loves full sun and poor, rocky soil. It is profuse in areas that have been razed or cleared—as if it congregates to heal these areas as soon as the land has been damaged. If cultivated, once it gets established, it's better not to fertilize or water it much. In fact, for a more medicinal effect from the harvest during the flowering stage, watering should be discontinued. This induced stress is similar to a wild plant's experience and seems to bring out more medicinal constituents.

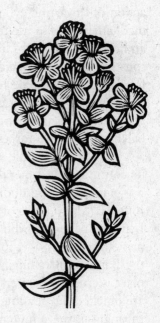

A Spiritual History

St. John's wort, *Hypericum perforatum*, grows in North and South America and Australia but is native to Europe where its history is rich. Derived from Greek, the name *Hypericum* means "over an apparition." Could this already be referring to its popular use today as a natural antidepressant? A midsummer herb, the Druids categorized it as a Sun-ruled plant. For the psyche and for spiritual matters, the Sun represented a strengthening influence toward cultivating a positive mind and fostering proactive, creative, and confident states. The Druids thought just a whiff of its balsamic, resinous scent was enough to repel evil forces and could dispel madness when used as medicine. Keep in mind, throughout much of history, people thought most illnesses were caused by evil spirits. Considering the whole of human history, only recently has science developed enough to offer us other explanations for diseases. This explains why, when reading about the historical use of herbs in numerous books, this extraordinary action of thwarting evil spirits is attributed to so many popular medicinal herbs in use today. The stronger the medicinal effect an herb has, the more likely you will read about it keeping bad spirits at bay. The Druids thought St. John's wort to be blessed for it contained the perfect balance of fire and water considered optimum for a healing effect. Fire was associated with the Sun and water associated with sinking into the dark, cold season. A balance of the two forces was Midsummer.

During the Middle Ages, use of this herb to banish evil spirits continued. In June, the plant begins flowering and a bundle was hung over the door and replaced every Summer Solstice, June 21. These kinds of Pagan activities were of concern to the Benedictine monks who then dignified the herb with a Christian name honoring Saint John's Day, June 24, the birthday of John the Baptist. "Bleeding" appears to happen when the flowering plant is crushed. Fingers are stained bright red when the flowers are pinched. Depending on the climate, flowering can continue throughout the summer, and in August it was thought the plant bled on the day John the Baptist was beheaded. Interestingly enough, we now know the plant is at its medicinal optimum when the flowering stage has progressed to the point when fruits and seeds begin to appear. Did they know August was an optimum time for making St. John's wort medicine? The ancient doctors of Rome and Greece associated its appearance of bleeding with its highly successful ability to heal wounds. Coincidentally (or not) in the 1600s, herbalist John Coles promoted the Doctrine of Signatures, which established connections between a plant's appearance and its ability to heal a particular condition. He suggested a connection between the tiny holes visible on a St. John's wort leaf when held up to the Sun and the pores of our skin. These little "holes" are actually glands also described as hypericin idioblasts, which contain the red pigments that also contribute to the mysterious bleeding effect. Coles recommended its use for "hurts and wounds and inward bruises." The species name, *perforatum*, is due to the impression of a leaf full of small holes.

Healing Oils

A healing oil was made by soaking or infusing the St. John's wort flowering tops into a vegetable oil such as olive oil. Infused oil such as this has been a staple of traditional herbal medicine since the beginning. The red pigments characteristic of this plant make a beautiful red oil. The herb material in the vegetable oil is usually allowed to infuse together (macerate) in a jar placed in a dark place for a few weeks. The sun seems to be the best place to set a jar of St. John's wort oil to bring out more of the flavonoids for healing and the constituent, hyperforin, known for antibacterial action. Modern explanations abound as to why the prepared oil is such a soothing dressing for sores, cuts, wounds, burns, hemorrhoids, varicose veins, bruises, ulcers, bites, and for both traumatic and chronic nerve pain due to injuries or surgery, arthritis, sciatica, lumbago, and neuralgia. Studies show remarkable success for healing first-, second-, and third-degree burns—

three times faster than normal and with less scarring. The power of St. John's wort to prevent and heal skin damage from radiation treatments has been empirically observed. Antibacterial action has even been clinically proven for staph infections.

Wound-Healing Tinctures and Teas

In addition to application of the healing oil, a study found that a traditionally prepared tincture of St. John's wort taken internally was superior to the topical application of calendula tincture for healing a wound. For the internal use of any herb to heal a wound better than a well-known topical remedy like calendula is remarkable. Studies have not been conducted for every known topical use of this herb, but modern use has demonstrated its ability to decrease nerve pain and repair nerve damage. Some resources are specific in referring to severed nerves, crushed fingers or limbs, sports injuries, and postsurgical pain. There are reports of dramatic pain relief experienced by wild-crafters of the herb after a few days of harvesting stained their hands of the medicinal compounds. After a few weeks of harvesting, one wild-crafter reported to be completely free of a long-standing, severe case of sciatica.

Taken internally as tea or in the extract/tincture form, St. John's wort helps many of the same painful conditions commonly treated externally with the oil. Obviously, its analgesic and anti-inflammatory effects are useful, but the fact that it is a sedative and nervine (tonic for the nervous system) must also play a role. Being more relaxed and less anxious definitely helps when coping with pain. Settling the nerves has also proved St. John's wort's usefulness for smoking cessation, during perimenopause and menopause, counteracting the stress of our modern lifestyle, panic, anxiety, and grief. Other historical uses have been as an astringent, which is an agent that contracts or tightens tissue. Astringents have traditionally been used for diarrhea or dysentery and, to a lesser extent, various digestive problems like nausea, ulcers, and gastritis.

Virus Vanquisher

Both internal and external preparations have proven to be exceptionally comforting to the various symptoms of viruses of the herpes family. The infused oil is a famous treatment to the blistered or painful areas resulting from the condition known as shingles, or herpes zoster. The analgesic, wound-healing, and antiseptic qualities are also in play for this application. Ingestion of the tea or extract is clearly suggested, but some sufferers get remarkable relief by pouring, spraying, or otherwise applying the tea to the affected areas. A clever method is to partially fill ice cube trays with the strong tea, freeze, and apply the "tea cubes" whenever desired. Cold sores and outbreaks of genital herpes are also treated with all the various external and internal St. John's wort products. Rare in the pharmaceutical kingdom are chemicals with an antiviral activity, but they are not rare in plant medicine. St. John's wort's antiviral action may also be why it is a supreme herpes remedy as well as a supportive preventative measure when taken internally between outbreaks.

Immunity Booster

HIV is a virus that causes AIDS and leaves the body defenseless against many other illnesses including respiratory, digestive, and herpes infections. Research using many of the constituents contained in St. John's wort is showing the ability to reduce the spread of HIV in a test tube. Specifically, hypericin and pseudohypericin are two of the many naturally occurring chemical constituents that inhibit herpes simplex types 1 and 2 and HIV type 1. While research continues, those in the herbal community see the obvious benefits of the basic antiviral, antibacterial, antidepressant, nerve-soothing, and immune-protecting qualities as reason enough to consider its use valuable when living with HIV. Interestingly, research has shown activity against a host of viruses including influenza, herpes, polio, HIV, and hepatitis C.

Antidepressant

A few words about antidepressants seem unavoidable when the topic happens to be St. John's wort. This herb has been proven to act as both a monoamine oxidase inhibitor, or MAOI (popular pharmaceutical brands are Marplan, Nardil, Parnate), and as a selective serotonin reuptake inhibitor, SSRI (Prozac, Luvox, and Zoloft). The standard caution about avoiding this herb use if taking these prescriptions sounds rather alarming. The fact behind this caution is that the herb enhances the power of the drug, or duplicates the activity. What this really means is that it makes good sense to work with your health professional to determine how much less pharmaceutical you will need in combination with use of the natural herb for the same effect. Considering that a pronounced lack of side effects was one of the featured outcomes after testing the herb on three thousand patients, incorporating St. John's wort in combination with pharmaceuticals is worth considering.

Illness is often accompanied by depression. Consider the usefulness of such an herb when the antidepressant benefits are well established, as are so many other benefits for combattingnerve problems, nervous system debility, and viral invaders present with chronic diseases like multiple sclerosis, post-herpetic neuralgia, arthritis, rheumatism, chronic fatigue syndrome, fibromyalgia, and HIV/AIDS.

The properties that relieve depression also have some crossover benefits. A connection between St. John's wort and Parkinson's has already been made. One explanation is the mild MAOI effect. Since the enzyme monoamine oxidase (MAO) suppresses dopamine, inhibiting MAOs can boost dopamine levels, which is believed to reduce the risk for Parkinson's. (This is the current assumption as to why this herb seems helpful for Parkinson's, but what about the value it presents to the nerves in general? Often a single herb follows many avenues of healing for one condition.)

Shining a Light on Side Effects

Exposure to sunlight is of some concern regarding the use of St. John's wort. Grazing animals that eat large amounts of this plant have become hypersensitive to the sun to the point of developing blistered skin. This resulted in warnings for humans consuming the plant to avoid prolonged exposure to sunlight. Ever watchful for upholding the highest integrity and level of safety, the medicinal herb industry encourages the notification of all known warnings with products. This particular warning continues to be published even though it has also been established that the dose required for a human to become photosensitized by St. John's wort would be thirty times higher than what is needed for its antidepressant effect. Normal use is not a concern regarding time spent in the sun. In fact, it's notable that topical use of the infused oil will speed the healing of any such burns. Another notable fact is the conclusion of a Canadian study showing that exposure to light was required for hypericin to inactivate the AIDS virus. Quite possibly anyone using this herb for HIV would be advised to spend a little time in the sunshine on a regular basis. Sunshine is often recommended for those suffering with depression and, of course, seasonal affective disorder (SAD).

We often associate the sun with things enjoyable and uplifting. Someone has a "sunny disposition" or someone "brings sunshine" into someone's life. St. John's wort's sunny, yellow, midsummer-blooming flowers represent the Sun quite well, which continues to encourage us to connect our use of the herb with the sun. The Druids considered it blessed for its perfect Midsummer balance but perhaps we are the ones blessed to have such a remarkable sunny herb.

For Further Reading

Castleman, Michael. *The New Healing Herbs*. Emmaus, Pennsylvania: Rodale Press, 2001.

Cech, Richo. *Herb of the Sun, Saint John's Wort*. Williams, Oregon: Horizon Herbs, 1997.

Cech, Richo. *Making Plant Medicine*. Williams, Oregon: Horizon Herbs. 2000.

Duke, James A. *Dr. Duke's Essential Herbs*. New York: St. Martin's Paperbacks. 2001.

Foster, Steven and Duke, James. *Peterson Field Guides, Eastern/Central Medicinal Plants*. Boston: Houghton Mifflin Company, 1990.

Hopman, Ellen Evert. *A Druid's Herbal for the Sacred Earth Year*. Rochester, Vermont: Destiny Books, 1995.

Kowalchik, Claire, and William Hylton, Ed. *Rodale's Illustrated Encyclopedia of Herbs*. Emmaus, Pennsylvania: Rodale Press, 1987.

Meyer, Joseph. *The Herbalist*. Glenwood, Illinois: Meyerbooks, 1960.

Treben, Maria. *Health through God's Pharmacy*. Steyr, Austria: Wilhelm Ennsthaler, 1991.

Upton, Roy. *St. John's Wort Hypericum perforatum*. Austin, Texas: American Botanical Council, 1998.

Wren, R.C. *Potter's New Cyclopaedia of Botanical Drugs & Preparations*. Saffron Walden: The C.W. Daniel Company Ltd. 1994.

The Healing Power of Comfrey

by Sue Morris

Comfrey—even the name evokes a comforting feeling—is a healing plant, often undervalued due to its persistent quality and abundant availability, yet treasured by herbalists for its well-regarded ability to heal chronic skin ailments, wounds, itchy rashes, and even broken bones.

Its botanical name, *Symphytum officinale*, comes from a Greek word meaning "to unite," and this plant's capacity to unite or regenerate skin tissue, heal broken bones, and take the discoloration out of a black-and-blue patch as well as rectify a multitude of other skin disorders is, I believe, second to none.

A leafy perennial with long, hairy leaves that will cause you to itch when touched, comfrey has bell-like purple flowers furling in clusters from the top of large hairy stems, and grows up to

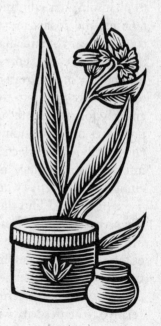

two to three feet high, flowering from early spring to summer. The roots are large and sturdy, spreading deeply and with great doggedness so as to not want to be removed from the earth once established. It will grow in sun or shade, but prefers the cool shade and does not have a need for high-quality soil. Comfrey is a fast-growing plant that produces huge amounts of leaves during the growing season, and hence is very nitrogen hungry. It appreciates manure applied as mulch, lawn clippings, and other nitrogen-rich materials but will grow without these quite well. Comfrey plants can be cut down several times a season and will re-grow, making it a wonderful plant to use throughout the spring, summer and well into fall.

It asks for very little and returns a great deal when used appropriately as needed.

The root is known for its glutinous and mucilaginous nature and is rich in allantoin, the compound known to promote tissue regeneration. Pharmacologically, the wound healing is attributed to allantoin, but comfrey also has pyrrolizidine alkaloids (Pas), tannins, and rosmarinic acid, a proven anti-inflammatory. Both root and leaf contain allantoin, but comfrey root contains about ten times the concentration of Pas found in the leaves. The internal use of comfrey is discouraged because of its alkaloid content, and according to the *Physicians' Desk Reference* "one should entirely forgo the internal administration of comfrey due to the presences of pyrrolizidine alkaloids (Pas) which have hepatotoxic and carcinogenic effects." In other words, do not take comfrey internally, for instance as a tea, as it has been shown to have carcinogenic properties when studied in male rats.

Personally, I find this interesting as "comfrey has been used since the sixteenth century for not only wound healing and inflammation, but also for treating gout, ulcers, diarrhea, dysentery, internal ulcers, bronchitis, mastitis, pleurisy, and fibrositis," according to Michelle Mairesse, author of *Health Secrets of Medicinal Herbs*. Futhermore, the effects are cumulative and "the relative toxicities vary widely depending on the part of the plant consumed and from one species to another of the same genus," according to Michael McGuffin, editor of the American Herbal Association's *Botanical Safety Handbook*.

Allantoin has been chemically synthesized by the cosmetic industry as an over-the-counter active ingredient in sun-care products, clarifying lotions, creams, anti-acne products, and oral-hygiene products such as toothpaste and mouthwashes. It is known for its moisturizing and keratolytic effect, meaning it increases the water content of the extracellular matrix of skin and enhances the removal of upper layers of dead skin cells, increasing the smoothness of skin and promoting wound healing; and a soothing, anti-irritant, and skin-protecting effect. The external uses are encouraged and undeniably potent.

Comfrey can also have a profound effect on our internal structure once we look beneath the surface. The roots of the plant are remarkable. Personally, I have been fascinated by their resemblance to the human anatomy—the older the root, the more like arms, legs, and pelvic bones it looks. As an astrologer and herbalist, I am an advocate of the system of "the Doctrine of Signatures," the medieval cosmology based on the concept that the inherent qualities of all things leave their mark, or "signature," on all animate and inanimate objects, in this case plants, therefore describing its healing benefit by the nature of its physical character. In the case of comfrey, a Saturn-ruled plant, the leaves resemble skin and the roots resemble bones. Comfrey delivers on its planetary connection as an effective remedy for skin, teeth, and bone ailments.

According to Culpeper, "the roots being outwardly applied, cure fresh wounds or cuts immediately, so powerful that if they be boiled with dissevered pieces of flesh in a pot, it will join them together again." Any plant that can regenerate skin tissue and help heal fresh scars, wounds, and bruises is one to place a high value on.

In my own experience, comfrey was very useful when I deeply punctured my hand (just below the thumb) with a chef's knife and was hurting too badly to drive myself to the hospital for stitches. First, I stopped the bleeding by holding my hand under cold water and then holding the skin tightly together with a butterfly bandage. Then I soaked first some freshly picked comfrey leaves in warm water and wrapped the moist leaves tightly over the bandage on my hand. I changed the fresh leaves three to four times each day for three to four days and was left with virtually no scarring at all. I had no need for stitches. I avoided using comfrey salve at first because I didn't want the top layer of skin to heal too quickly, as the wound was deep. The comfrey leaves helped speed up the cell proliferation that enabled the wound to heal quickly.

The comfrey salve I have created has healed a great variety of skin ailments, from chronic eczema, itchy rashes, scleroderma to fresh scars after surgery, scabs, scrapes, and bruises with almost immediate results. Two of the most grateful users of my comfrey salve firmly convinced me of the salve's efficacy.

The first was a man whom I met while I was selling my salves at a festival. He had a severe burn on his hand from an accident that occurred when he was working on a car. The car was on a lift and began to fall and his response was to reach up and stop it from falling on him. His hand came in contact with an extremely hot exhaust pipe and caused a severe burn that resulted in deep, unhealed cracks, which made even opening and closing his hand quite painful. He showed me the hand and said he'd tried everything on it, a multitude of prescription medications, lotions, and creams. I encouraged him to try a little salve on it, if for nothing more than to take away the dryness. He reluctantly and suspiciously put some on and walked away. About an hour later he returned, holding out both hands and asking "which one?" He said after using the salve only a few times his hand was so much better that you couldn't tell the burned one from the good one. He had suffered the pain and discomfort from that injury for over eight years!

The second most grateful person who used my comfrey salve was an eighty-year-old woman who sent me a testimonial after an ordeal with her scalp. She described herself as becoming severely depressed after a long period of time with a scalp condition. She wrote that she had a longstanding reputation for her beautiful, thick, and curly hair, "the healthiest hair even after forty years of dying my jet black tresses." It all changed when she developed a bad scalp problem, psoriasis all over her head. "Nothing I used seemed to help. Therapeutic shampoos made it worse, my hair stopped growing and my scalp became very itchy. "I applied Sue's salve one night before I went to bed and must report that almost immediately the condition disappeared completely!"

Many sufferers of chronic eczema have had wonderful results with my comfrey salves, particularly the tea tree salve, after years of prescription medications which they all have said did nothing to relieve the itchiness or rashes which they had. The comfrey salve in my line of Sue's Salves, contains both the leaf and root of the comfrey plant, as well as other healing plants such as fresh calendula flowers and fresh, whole aloe vera leaves. It has successfully treated such a variety of skin disorders and chronic skin problems and its efficacy continues to amaze everyone who uses it.

The power of plant healing is undeniable. Using the right plant for the right condition is the key to natural healing. There are many medicinal herbs that can be used to treat specific ailments and consulting an herbalist or researching the safety and appropriate medicinal uses is always recommended before using any plants. Mistaken identity is a possible cause of plant misuse, such as deadly nightshade leaves being mistaken for comfrey by inexperienced collectors of plants, or digitalis poisoning resulting in mistaking foxglove for comfrey.

Using fresh, organically grown healing herbs that are identified as safe is an effective and affordable way to benefit medicinally from the plant kingdom. As a plant lover and maker of natural skin-care remedies, I have been convinced time and time again of their effectiveness and safety when used properly.

When crafting Sue's Salves, I use only freshly harvested plants grown organically in my central Pennsylvania garden. Harvested according to the system of The Doctrine of Signatures, I carefully choose the planetary hour appropriate for the specific plant, i.e. the hour of Saturn (for example, the first two hours after dawn on Saturday) to harvest comfrey—as this is considered the peak of the plant's of potency. I steep the fresh plants in pure olive oil, strain them, and add fresh beeswax to create potent, healing skin salves that can treat maladies ranging from topical skin ailments from simple dry skin (when used as a face moisturizer) to such chronic skin disorders as chronic eczema and psoriasis and undiagnosed rashes, bruises, cold sores, cracked skin, sunburn, athlete's foot, and diaper rash. I add essential oils to my salves for their healing qualities, such as lavender for burns, peppermint for the feet, tea tree for fungal infections, and ylang ylang for a sensual and relaxing massage.

Comfrey is a plant that reminds me that natural healing is a simple and reverent process. Nature enables everyone to benefit from the healing qualities the plants so willingly offer. In return, all we must do is make careful use of what Mother Nature provides and return to her our gratitude by treating the Earth with gentle kindness and an appreciation of and respect for the botanical world. The animal kingdom has relied on the plant world for its survival and we will continue to do so until the end of time.

Gastrointestinal Health

❧ by Dallas Jennifer Cobb ❧

We are all aware of the importance of good health, but how many of us really know how to cultivate health in the area we are embarrassed to talk about—the deep, dark bowels? There is a growing incidence of conditions affecting the gastrointestinal tract and chronic disease. To help prevent and treat these conditions, understanding what the gastrointestinal tract is and how it works is essential.

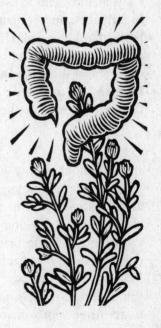

The gastrointestinal tract (or GI tract) is the system that breaks down and digests food, absorbing the nutrients our bodies need and discarding the waste material. With the mouth as the opening, the gastrointestinal tract is made up of the esophagus, a ten-inch tube that leads to the stomach—a densely muscled organ about the size of your fist. Following that is twenty feet of small intestine and six feet of large intestine, which is also called the colon. The end of the gastrointestinal tract is the rectum, where waste is excreted.

Problems that develop in the gastrointestinal tract range from so-called minor ailments like constipation and diarrhea to serious ailments like diverticulitis, irritable bowel syndrome, and colorectal cancer. About 70 million people in the United States are affected by gastrointestinal problems.

An understanding of how the organs in the gastrointestinal tract work can help prevent and treat ailments, and teach us how to help, rather than hinder, their functions.

For many years I suffered from constipation and bowel toxicity and found that none of the variety of prescriptions and medical procedures administered really resolved my condition. Finally, I started to research how my gastrointestinal tract worked, understanding what aggravated it, and what facilitated good function—for me.

The information listed here is a summary of my learning and experiences, and contains information on dietary changes and herbs that helped me. Like most any regimen, what worked for me might not work (or be safe) for you. For the safe and effective use of herbs please consult a chartered herbalist or naturopath for diagnosis and treatment of any ailments. With their guidance you may come to use herbal remedies with great success.

How It Works

It takes about twenty-four hours for a healthy gastrointestinal tract to process matter, from the time of eating to the time of waste elimination. For the average person, this process is considerably slower, taking up to four days.

Chewing is the first step in the process, as food is broken down through mastication and mixed with saliva. This slurry of food is swallowed down the esophagus, and passes into the stomach, where it is drenched in hydrochloric acid and turns into a paste. After approximately forty minutes, the paste travels into the small intestine, where nutrients are absorbed and delivered to the bloodstream. Further down, the large intestine, or colon, absorbs all of the remaining liquid and turns the paste into denser fecal matter. It then takes from one to four days for the fecal matter to twist its way through the colon before it is released as a bowel movement.

The average human carts around between five and seven pounds of waste in their system at any given time.

Healthy Bowel Habits

Because of an increased consumption of processed foods, a lower ingestion of fiber, and the development of subsequent gastrointestinal problems, we have come to think that if we have one bowel movement a day we are doing well. However, there is the "matter in, matter out" theory, which asserts that a healthy human should have a bowel movement about as often as they eat. So if you eat three large meals a day, you should have three large bowel movements per day.

Bowel movements should be expelled easily, without effort, waiting, or strain. They should be about one-foot long (up to about two feet) with a gentle curved shape similar to the intestines, and float in the bowl. It is common for the bowel to move every morning to expel waste from the prior day. This bowel movement will be considerably larger than others through the day because of the amount of matter that has been processed overnight.

When it is necessary to strain, push, or wait for the bowel to move, or if the stool is small, narrow, short, or hard, the bowel is not functioning correctly. Other indications of poor bowel function include seeing mucus, blood, or half-digested food in the stool. But don't be alarmed by occasionally seeing certain difficult-to-digest foods like corn or peas in your stool.

How To Help the Bowel

Following some simple guidelines for healthy bowel activity can increase both the frequency and volume of bowel movements, effectively ridding the body of its waste materials. These guidelines include drinking eight to ten glasses of water per day, eating primarily whole foods in their whole state, avoiding processed foods, and consuming at least ten servings of fruits and vegetables each day.

Because of the widespread availability of fast foods, processed foods, and snack items, many of us don't reach even the minimum dietary guidelines for healthy bowel function.

When we follow these simple guidelines, bowel activity becomes regular and frequent, eliminating a large volume of waste material. The small intestine isn't hampered and can easily absorb the needed nutrients, and the large intestine is unencumbered, able to effectively absorb water, and easily release waste materials.

Common Bowel Problems

Constipation

While we often talk about constipation as a common, harmless condition, constipation is more serious than we have been lead to believe. Constipation is primarily due to poor diet. Generally considered to be anything that slows the eliminatory system down, constipation contributes to buildup in the digestive and eliminatory tract, causing greater systemic toxicity and discomfort. With lowered levels of fiber and water in the diet, food is slower to process. By the time it reaches the large intestine, it is already a sticky mass that moves very slowly. As the large intestine continues to remove water from the matter, it creates dense, dry, and compacted fecal matter that can literally sit in the colon for days.

With the slowed processing of matter comes putrefaction, the decomposition of organic matter by microorganisms (or rotting), of food. This putrefied material sits in the small and large intestine where it creates irritation or inflammation. In response to the irritation, the small and large intestines produce mucus to soothe the irritated membranes. This mucus lines the intestines to protect them. If the irritation is a temporary condition the mucus lining is no longer needed and is often eliminated in the fecal matter once the irritation has passed.

Chronic constipation, when the irritating conditions persist, is a result of habitual poor diet and bad eating habits. Bowel movements become infrequent and difficult to pass because of dry, tightly compacted fecal matter. With chronic constipation, the protective mucous lining is never shed from the intestines, and gets thicker and gooier over time. With the removal of water the mucous lining becomes dehydrated and harder, achieving a consistency similar to tire rubber, which is very difficult to get rid of.

This dried feces combined with the accumulated mucus adheres to the walls of the colon in a tarlike mass. This makes the small intestine's usual function of nutrient absorption much more difficult and increases the chances that toxins produced by the built up matter are absorbed into the bloodstream.

Chronic constipation also causes a variety of other problems. The compacted matter is an ideal environment for harboring parasites, bacteria, and infection.

Herbs to Help Constipation

The primary cause of constipation is diet, so undertaking dietary improvement would be the first practical step. The guidelines for good bowel function, as stated above, include eight to ten glasses of water per day, eating a variety of whole foods in their whole state, and consuming ten fruits and/or vegetables per day.

Herbs that help heal constipation fall into three categories: bulk or high-fiber herbs, laxatives, and purgatives. Bulk or high fiber herbs simply provide additional fiber to sweep through the system, cleansing and removing built-up waste. Laxative herbs help to relax the bowels, loosening matter and facilitating evacuation. Purgative herbs purge the bowels, usually by stimulating bowel contractions.

The safest herbs recommended for use by those experiencing constipation are those with a high fiber or bulk content such as:

- Flaxseed (also known as linseed) (*Linum usitatissimum*)
- Psyllium (*Plantago psyillium*)
- Fenugreek (*Trigonella foenum-graecum*)

Avoid herbs that are considered laxatives or purgatives. These herbs don't facilitate the natural function of the bowels, but instead stimulate bowel function unnaturally. They can cause the bowels to contract spasmodically and create messy situations if you lose control of the bowels. Prolonged use of laxatives and purgatives can also create "lazy bowel syndrome" in which the bowel forgets how to function normally, becoming reliant on outside stimulation.

Many of the purgative herbs are also considered to be irritants and are unsafe for pregnant or nursing women, as well as people with gastrointestinal problems like ulcers, irritable bowel syndrome, and hemorrhoids.

Parasites

While often associated with Third World countries, parasites in developed countries are more common than you think. The type of parasites that humans can play host to are varied and numerous, from microscopic to enormous tapeworms several feet long. In North America, amoebas such as Giardia (which causes giardiasis, a.k.a. Beaver Fever) and pinworms are common causes of intestinal infections. Roundworm, whip worm, hookworm, and schistosomes are all common culprits.

Parasites are contracted through contaminated water, undercooked meats, and unwashed fruits and vegetables. They are also transmitted from pets or livestock. Parasites can reside in almost any part of the body but are most common in the colon. The moist, dark environment with lots of food and putrefied material is an ideal habitat. Maintaining good intestinal flora can raise the body's natural resistance to parasites, while overuse of antibiotics lowers the resistance by killing off helpful intestinal flora.

Herbs to Heal Parasites

Talk to your health care practitioner, preferably a chartered herbalist, before using herbs to treat parasites. A sound diagnosis is essential before any treatment is prescribed. Many herbs used to treat parasites are powerful, and in some cases have toxic side effects. What will be prescribed depends on the type of parasite, your current state of health, and other lifestyle factors. Many of these herbs are not advised for pregnant or lactating women or people with other gastrointestinal problems.

Lactobacillus acidophillus, the culture commonly used to make yogurt, is one of the most widely used probiotics known to humans. To keep your gut in good shape and naturally resistant to parasites, add probiotics to your diet by consuming either a good quality yogurt with live culture or taking supplements.

Herbs to heal parasites come in two types, depending on their qualities: vermifuge or vermicide. A vermifuge flushes the worms out of the system, and a vermicide kills the worms. One of the greatest combined vermifuge and vermicide is garlic (*Allium sativum*), which both kills the parasite and flushes it out of the system. Why not add garlic to your diet in its raw and cooked state for flavor, improved immunity, and parasite-fighting functions?

Herbs commonly used to treat parasites include:

Aloe vera (*Aloe socotrina*)
Anise (*Pimpinella anisum*
Barberry (*Berberis vulgaris*)
Black walnut husk (*Juglans nigra*)
Garlic (*Allium sativum*)
Goldenseal (*Hydrastis canadensis*)
Curled mint (*Mentha crispa*)
Oregon grape (*Berberis aquifolium*)
Tea tree oil (*Melaleuca alternifolia*)
Wormwood (*Artemisia annua*)
Yellow dock (*Rumex crispus*)

In tropical countries, people commonly drink aloe vera gel mixed with lime juice three times a day for three days following mango season. Mangoes commonly harbor parasites, so people take a "wash out" afterward to get rid of the parasites. Because aloe vera is powerful and causes bowel contractions, it is not recommended for everyone and should never be used on a long-term basis.

Diverticulosis and Diverticulitis

When dried fecal matter compacts in the colon it can cause the development of small pouches or bulges called diverticuli. These pouches form because of the pressure created both by the compacted matter and the gases that escape from the putrefaction process. This condition is diverticulosis, and it is quite common in North America. About 30 percent of adult North Americans and over half of those over the age of forty have diverticulosis.

When the pouches or bulges become infected or inflamed, the condition progresses to be called diverticulitis, the condition of chronic infection and irritation of the lining of the intestinal wall. Not only is the condition painful, but it contributes to systemic toxicity and malabsorbtion of vitamin B12, an essential vitamin. In severe cases, diverticulitis causes the bowel to rupture—a life-threatening condition.

Herbs to Help Diverticulosis

Diverticulosis and diverticulitis are associated with a poor diet that relies heavily on meat and processed foods. The first line of treatment is dietary—considerably increasing fiber and water. With increased fiber in the diet the intracolic pressure (pressure needed to expel a bowel movement) decreases. This reduces the chances of herniation or pocket formation due to pressure or straining.

Herbs that increase fiber or bulk can help, such as:

Flaxseed (also known as linseed) (*Linum usitatissimum*)
Psyllium (*Plantago psyillium*)
Fenugreek (*Trigonella foenum-graecum*)

Other commonly used herbs include those that heal and tonify the intestinal wall, such as:

Cascara sagrada or 'Sacred Grass' (*Rhamnus purshiana*)
Alfalfa (*Medicago sativa*)
Hibiscus flower (*Hibiscus sabdariffa*)
Licorice root (*Glycyrrhiza glabra*)
Slippery elm bark (*Ulmus rubra*)

Irritable Bowel Syndrome

Spasms of the intestine causing nausea, bloating, discomfort, and cramps are lumped together under the name irritable bowel syndrome. IBS is experienced by over 20 percent of adults. While many of us have been lead to think that it is caused by a malfunction of the nerves that control the intestine, it is more likely a symptom of bowel toxicity.

Irritable bowel syndrome is best treated through an increase in dietary fiber, the cultivation of healthy intestinal flora, and the reduction of bowel toxicity through improved bowel function. Herbs to relieve constipation and heal inflamed tissues are cited above.

Diarrhea

While diarrhea seems to be the opposite of constipation, both diarrhea and constipation are caused by the same things: fecal encrustation and bowel toxicity. Trying to defend itself against toxins, the body flushes water into the colon in an attempt to wash out the waste. Prolonged diarrhea causes dehydration because fluids are pulled from other bodily tissues.

How to Heal Diarrhea

If the colon is clean and functioning well, there is no reason to flush it out. By improving the diet, increasing dietary fiber and drinking lots of water, we enable the colon to function normally, ridding itself of fecal matter and toxins.

Preventing Toxic Buildup

Almost all afflictions of the gastrointestinal tract are a combination of autointoxication (when the body becomes toxic and forces the blood system to absorb toxic materials) and malnutrition (as a result of the lack of available nutrients). The combination of high levels of toxins plus poor levels of absorbed nutrients leave the body vulnerable to the ill effects of many toxic compounds that are byproducts of autointoxication, such as:

- ammonia and amines, which are liver toxins
- nitrosamines, indoles, and skatoles, which are known carcinogens (meaning they cause cancer)
- phenols and cresols, which promote cancer and facilitate cancerous growth
- estrogens, which are suspected carcinogens heavily linked to the development of breast cancer
- secondary bile acids, which are carcinogenic and promote colon cancer
- aglycones, which are mutagenic organisms

When you review a list like this it is easy to understand the disastrous, and often fatal, secondary effects of gastrointestinal illnesses. However, the easiest way to heal gastrointestinal problems (and to prevent them) is to stop doing things that hamper bowel function, and start doing things that help it. Things that hamper bowel function include:

- a diet low in fiber
- eating too many processed foods
- not drinking enough fluids
- inactivity

So try to eliminate foods that lead to constipation like white flour, processed foods, and dairy products. Avoid sticky foods like sugar, sweets, and hydrogenated oils. Stay away from low water content foods like pasta, baked goods, and breads.

Eating fiber-rich whole foods is a great way to help keep the GI system moving. Foods that are high in dietary fire include all fruits and vegetables, legumes, whole grains, and raw nuts and seeds. Such a high-fiber diet will help to cleanse the bowels and eliminate toxic buildup. While it takes a long time to clean out old built-up matter, a diet rich in fiber will eventually scrub out the intestines, and start to empty out the pockets of diverticuli. As long as you are not adding to the toxic burden, you are contributing to the health and proper functioning of your bowels.

Beyond diet, the one thing that most aids the bowels in their normal functioning is bowel cleansing. This can be done with assistance through enemas and other colon cleansing techniques, or naturally by increasing dietary fiber.

Herbal Formulas

A wide variety of herbal formulas available are marketed as promoting good bowel and digestive health. While I will not endorse any specific companies or formulas, leaving that to your chartered herbalist or naturopath, I will note that the vast majority of them include many bulk herbs, some laxative herbs, and a small amount of purgative herbs. Most of the following herbs are common in many of the "recipes":

Alfalfa (*Medicago sativa*)
Black walnut hulls (*Juglans nigra*)
Cascara sagrada or 'Sacred Grass' (*Rhamnus purshiana*)
Hibiscus flower (*Hibiscus sabdariffa*)
Irish moss (*Chondrus crispus*)
Licorice root (*Glycyrrhiza glabra*)
Marshmallow root (*Althaea officinalis*)
Mullein (*Verbascum thapsus*)
Oatstraw (*Avena sativa*)
Passionflower (*Passiflora incarnata*)
Psyllium (*Plantago ovata*)
Pumpkin seeds (*Cucurbita pepo*)

Shavegrass (*Equisetum arvense*)
Slippery elm bark (*Ulmus rubra*)
Stevia (*Stevia rebaudiana*)
Violet (*Viola odorata*)
Witch hazel (*Hamamelis virginiana*)
Yucca (*Yucca schidigera/Yucca brevifolia*)

Whatever our health ailments, a focus on gastrointestinal health and the health of our bowels will have positive results. Eliminating toxic residue from the colon can result in weight loss, improved nutrient absorption, reduced toxins in the system, and an overall improvement in the functioning of all our vital organs.

So when you start to think about improving your health, start with the basics: eight to ten glasses of water per day, lots of fruits and vegetables, a whole foods diet, and lots of gentle activity. When they are needed, herbs provide a strong natural addition to the foundation established and will help to treat minor ailments and prevent illness.

Natural Remedies for Our Animal Companions

≈ by Krystal Bowden ≈

Those of us who try to live a healthier, nontoxic lifestyle, whether by using herbal remedies or avoiding harsh household chemicals, also want our animal companions to reap the benefits as well. While far fewer resources exist about natural health for animals, there are many simple things we can do using herbs to help our animal companions.

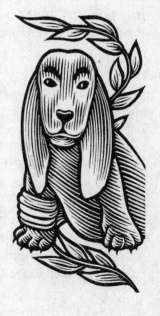

Remember that dogs, cats, and animals in general have a much stronger sense of smell than humans. Only a small amount of essential oils is needed to be effective; this is especially true for the animals in our care. Animals also have a sense of what is good for them; if they seem unhappy with a certain oil, try another one with a similar effect. If the new oil isn't satisfactory, take the time to double-check that you've properly identified the problem.

Fleas and Ticks

For those of us who love dogs and cats, our greatest fears for them can be fleas and ticks. Flea collars and store-bought drops tend to be less effective than we would like and can expose our animal friends to toxic chemicals. Our best natural defense for our dog is to give her a bath with peppermint castile soap. We rarely have a problem with any sort of bug, as the peppermint acts as a repellent for fleas and ticks. You can also try making your own flea collar using the following recipe: take a soft, natural-material collar (or make one yourself) and mix one drop each of essential oils of cedarwood, lavender, citronella, and thyme. Drop the mixture evenly around the collar. It should last about a month. Keep additional mixture in a bottle with a dropper as an easy way to refresh the collar. You will only need about four drops each time depending on your dog's size. Add a drop if your dog is particularly large or use only three drops for tiny dogs. You can also put a drop of the mixture on the brush when you groom them—it gives their coat a nice shine while preventing fleas. Some people swear by adding garlic to their pets' diets during the spring and summer, so it's worth a try. If flea drops are needed, though, it's better to get them from your veterinarian than to buy them at the store.

Cuts and Scrapes

For cuts and scrapes, what works on people generally works for animals. Bathe the area often using a half-gallon of water with one drop each of lavender and tea tree essential oils. Keep the area clean. For infected or ulcerous wounds, use a wilted cabbage leaf as a compress and change it several times a day. The cabbage leaves draw out the fluids that cause swelling and inflammation. Once the swelling has gone down, bathe the wound with the lavender and tea tree mixture. Try to keep it covered, and watch it closely for signs of further infection. This remedy also works for ear cankers. For minor burns, use one drop of lavender in two cups of very cold water and bathe the area as often as possible.

Warm wilted cabbage leaves can also help alleviate the pain of arthritis and other joint ailments in older animals. Take a single leaf and either iron it or put in the microwave or a warm oven for five to ten seconds until it is wilted, then gently cover the affected area. If necessary, you can wrap a sterile bandage around the area to keep the leaf in place. You can also try a massage using two drops of lavender in two teaspoons of carrier oil. Use short, gentle strokes going toward the heart. Be sure to massage through the coat to the joint, and treat the animal with respect: Don't wake him or her up to give a massage—follow their cues, be very gentle, and stop when they are ready for you to stop. Some animals get very nervous at unfamiliar occurrences, so it may take a few tries before your animal companion realizes you are trying to help.

Our Feline Friends

Many people love cats but hate what they do to the furniture. Cats need to have something available to scratch to sharpen and prevent overgrowth of their claws, even if you trim them on a regular basis. You can take a piece of wood (just about anything will do that they can brace themselves on) and either leave it plain or wrap it with hemp rope or dye-free leather and soak it in a strong infusion of catnip. Or put the infusion in a spray bottle and spray it on the scratching board. Another way to make a scratching board that is a bit more involved is to take heavyweight cardboard scraps and cut them to uniform size, about 2 by 24 inches. You will need about 20 to 25 of these strips. Lay the long sides of the strips of cardboard alongside each other, like books on a shelf, so that the inner layer of the cardboard (the wavy part) is facing up. Apply nontoxic glue between each of the layers (on the long side) and allow to dry. You will end up with a scratching post that is about 24 inches long, 2 inches high, and 6 inches wide. Spray it with catnip infusion, or sprinkle a few of the leaves on top. (This is basically how those disposable scratching posts you can buy at stores are made, so if you have a sturdy box lying around, it is cheaper to make one at home.) You may have to show the new scratching area to the cat, but they usually get the hang of it very quickly. If you still have a problem with cats scratching the furniture, try spraying the trouble spots with a mixture if one cup of water and four drops of orange essential oil (spot check a small area first). Some cats are repelled by orange oil and some are not, but it is worth a try to see if it works with your cat.

Other Animals

Spreading dried herbs on the bottom of smaller pens or cages, such as for rabbits or hamsters, can help keep them healthier and happier. Lavender is a good choice; the animals seem to like it, and it helps prevent flies and other insects from breeding. Wash out cages with a drop each of lavender and eucalyptus in a half-gallon of water.

For any animal that lives in a stall or pen, insects and/or rodents can be a problem. Mice have a particular aversion to peppermint, so try putting a drop of this essential oil in each corner of the stall, or add ten drops to one gallon of water to use as a rinse after the area has been otherwise cleaned. Other oils that repel rodents are spearmint, patchouli, and garlic. If insects are a problem, try one or two of the following: patchouli, tea tree, lavender, lemongrass, citronella, thyme, or peppermint. These can be used a few drops at a time around the stall and stable area, and will also keep the bugs away from anyone else in the area!

And finally, a few tips that don't fit anywhere else: If your horse is being bothered by flies or other insects, add two or three drops of lemongrass or lavender essential oil to their soft brush just before you brush them down. To increase and/or improve milk production in goats or cows, try adding fennel to their feed. Avoid using parsley or peppermint around milk animals, as this can decrease their milk production.

Our animal companions need and deserve the same care as their caretakers. If you have any questions or problems, do not hesitate to call your veterinarian.

Pet Food Cooked with Love (and Herbs)

≫ by Kaaren Christ ≪

As parents, we recognize that the time we spend planning and preparing food for our children is both a responsibility and an emotionally satisfying event. The energy we put into these tasks ensures our children receive a wide variety of high-quality, healthy food that is also appealing in appearance, smell, and taste.

Like our children, dog and cat companions are also members of our families. They too are almost solely dependent on us to help them enjoy rich day-to-day lives. With a desire to see our pets happy, we play, scratch, pet, groom, and exercise them daily. Above all else, we provide the healthy food they require to get the nutrition needed to live long healthy lives.

But what food is best? You will find countless varieties of dry kibble and

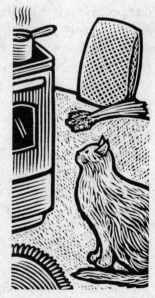

canned food in grocery store aisles and at the veterinary office that offer as wide a range of substance as price. However, many people are turning to a more balanced, wholesome approach to feeding their pets.

With the recent concerns about the lack of regulation for commercially produced pet foods, many people are finding a wonderful sense of satisfaction in learning to make their pet's food right at home. In addition to choosing the meats, fish, carbohydrates, and vegetables that will make up their furry friend's diet, they are also able to use herbs to further enhance the food.

What Do Dogs and Cats 'Need'?

Cats and dogs are different, so the way we feed them at home needs to reflect that. Our feline friends are carnivores and must eat meat in order to survive. Dogs are a little different in that they are classified as omnivores and can survive on either a plant or meat diet. Most sources caution against a fully vegetarian diet because it is difficult to offer the necessary variety to make it nutritionally balanced. In addition, dietary requirements can vary among breeds, so it's important to research the specific requirements of your pet before beginning to cook for them.

Generally, home-cooked pet meals should contain quality protein sources (meats and fish) as the primary ingredient, a balance of carbohydrates (cooked rice, potatoes, and grains), and fats and fiber. You can also mix in a variety of herbs to assist with repelling fleas, calming digestion, and treating motion sickness.

Benefits of Home Cooking

Pet owners who cook for their pets will tell you that this is the number one benefit of cooking homemade meals: "It's fun!" After that, they offer a host of other reasons. Some say they appreciate the low cost; others explain how it offers peace of mind to know what is going in their pet's mouths. Some value how it enhances the relationship they have with their animal companion, who sits patiently at their feet while they stir the pot. Still others say that since changing to home-cooked food, their pet's sensitive skin has improved or their hyperactive pet is more relaxed. Many also find it very satisfying to use herbal remedies in the same way we do for ourselves.

Home-Cooked Quality

We are turning back to Mother Nature for instruction on healthy eating and nutrition. After decades of focusing on convenience, there is a growing trend to return to simple, unprocessed food for our families. People who make home-cooked meals for pets point out that science has shown human beings to be healthier and live longer when they eat a diet of mostly natural, unprocessed foods. This is because the manufacturing process foods go through reduces its nutritional value.

The same principle applies for our dog and cat friends. In addition to the manufacturing process, there are also additives and preservatives added to manufacturers' foods which may be unhealthy for our pet. On the contrary, home-cooked meals lack the byproducts, preservatives, food coloring, and other chemicals found in manufactured food. When we have researched the nutritional needs of our companions and know that what they are being fed is wholesome, healthy, and additive- and preservative-free, we feel a peace of mind knowing we are giving our friends excellent care. A happy, healthy pet makes us feel good.

The Great Debate

People who cook for their pets usually feed them in one of two ways: with home-cooked food or "BARF" (which refers to "bones and raw food"). There seems to be a great debate waging as to which of these is more beneficial to the animal, and it certainly won't be decided here. Both have benefits and potential shortfalls, but ultimately, each animal lover will choose what they feel is best for their pet. In fact, some pet owners like to feed a mix of both. This decision is based on a range of factors; breed of animal, weight, health issues, age, and the preferences of both owner and animal. What works for one cat or dog won't always work for another—just like children. Furthermore, home-cooking does not have to be a full-time proposition. Pet lovers who aren't ready to start stirring the pot for their furry friends on a regular basis may enjoy making special dog or cat treats such as biscuits for rewards or a special meal on holidays.

Cost

Many people haven't considered cooking for their pets because they assume it is too costly. This, however, isn't usually the case. Purchasing ingredients in bulk will reduce the cost, which can be further decreased by sharing larger purchases with a friend. Proper storage of homemade food can minimize wasting any food by increasing the time it can be safely kept.

The Healthful Addition of Herbs

There are almost as many herbal remedies available for your pet as are available to you! Many can be added directly to food and others can be fed directly if your animal will accept it. Some herbs of particular interest include garlic, parsley, sage, peppermint, and red clover.

Garlic, in modest amounts, can be added to your pet's food for its antibacterial, antifungal, and antiviral properties. Garlic will help your pet's immune system and stimulate the liver and the colon, helping to rid the body of toxins. Parsley, most often used as a remedy for bad breath, can be sprinkled on food or baked into biscuits. Some pets can even be enticed to eat it raw out of your hands. Sage strengthens your pet's ability to concentrate and helps heal sores and remove dandruff. It's also popular for helping with digestive problems. Peppermint will tackle a bad case of flatulence and also relieve stress. Red clover is often used to help older animals heal from illness or injury.

Be Careful!

Make sure you research what is healthy and unhealthy for your dog or cat to eat before you begin. Dogs, for instance, should never be fed cooked bones because they might be brittle and could cause splinters in their stomachs. Certain foods can also make your dog sick. These include onions, avocado, grapes, chocolate, and mushrooms. Consult your veterinarian for a more complete list.

No matter which combinations of food you ultimately decide on, the time invested in cooking for your pet is time spent nurturing your relationship with your animal friend. They will appreciate the aroma of their meals on the stove and will come to recognize when you are cooking for them. You will feel appreciated, and your pet will be thrilled.

Recipes for Your Canine Friend

Three Bark Casserole

2 cups boiled and chopped chicken

1 cup cooked brown rice

1 teaspoon sage

1 cup boiled mixed vegetables (or any vegetable)

¼ cup unsalted chicken broth

Simply stir all ingredients together, sprinkle with fresh parsley, and serve at room temperature. (Salmon may sometimes be used instead of chicken, with chicken broth removed.) Put leftovers in a covered container in the refrigerator, where they will keep for three days.

Liver Biscuits

½   cup dry milk

½   cup wheat germ

1   teaspoon honey

½   cup homemade blended liver (or two jars of
       baby-food liver)

1   teaspoon garlic

1   teaspoon peppermint

Combine dry milk and wheat germ. Drizzle the honey on top. Add the liver, garlic, and peppermint.

Form the mixture into balls and bake at 200 degrees F. on a cookie sheet for 8 to 10 minutes. Consistency is slightly chewy. (Best served when your canine friend has rewarded you with generous wags and kisses.)

Treats for Your Mouser

Feline Hash

Simply stir together 1 cup cooked ground beef, ½ cup cooked brown rice, 6 teaspoons alfalfa sprouts, and ¾ cup cream-style cottage cheese. Place in fancy dish; set on special place.

Treats from the Sea

1   egg yolk

1   small trout fillet

3   tablespoons oatmeal

1   tablespoon vegetable oil

1   teaspoon parsley

Preheat the oven to 350 degrees F. Beat the egg and add finely chopped parsley to it. Dip the fish in the mixture and coat it with oatmeal. Place on baking sheet. Bake 15 minutes each side. Allow to cool. Cut into bite-sized pieces.

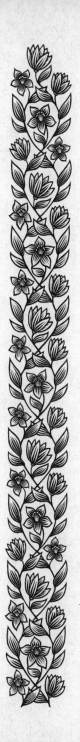

Herbs
for
Beauty

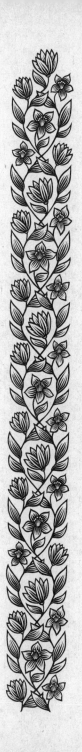

Herbal Care, Healthy Hair

❦ by Krystal Bowden ❦

Our hair is an integral part of who we are; it is one of the first things other people notice about us and perhaps our most identifying feature. It is a reflection of our general health and how we view ourselves. It gives others clues about our personality. We do all manner of things to make our hair look like we want it to—dye it, perm it, straighten it, gel and mousse it in a search (or, if we've found it, maintenance) of our ideal "look." The various chemicals in commercial products can be ultimately damaging, leading to the purchase of even more chemical-laden products to solve the problems caused by other chemicals—a vicious cycle. General hair health is also affected by diet and exercise, swimming, dyeing, perming—even by the amount of pollution in the air. I remember well the first

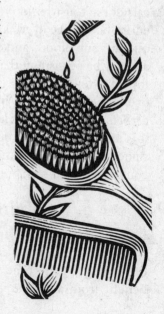

time I spent the night at a friend's house in the city. I woke up the next morning and wondered what had happened! My hair had gone from bright and clean to dull, lanky, and heavy in the course of a single night.

There are hundreds, if not thousands, of products designed for various aspects of hair care. Most contain a mix of chemicals with little study of how their long-term use might affect us. Quite a few of these chemicals are added to make the product aesthetically pleasing, such as dyes, perfumes, foaming/lathering enhancers, and anti-separation agents. Many of them now claim to be "all natural" or to contain "botanicals" or "herbal extracts," but often there is not a significant difference in the amount of chemicals nor is there more than a very tiny amount of recognizable botanicals. Check the label of your hair products—you may be surprised.

It's important to note that herbs don't just smell good, they have specific properties that can make your hair healthier overall. Herbs are absorbed into the body or skin, do their job, and leave our bodies gently. Using hair products with a lot of chemicals doesn't just harm your hair—they can cause stress to your entire body. The liver has to work harder to filter the chemicals out of your blood, and some of the artificial ingredients can actually be persistent; that is, they just stick around in your body for an extended time. These can have subtle effects on your overall health. We live in such a chemical-laden society—from carpets to clothing to cleaning products and many more—that it is important to limit our exposure to potentially harmful substances. This is most important with anything that comes into contact with our skin.

Tailor to Your Type

It is very beneficial to make your own hair products based on your hair type. They can be very simple or quite elaborate depending on the time you have available. All hair types will benefit from a simple vinegar rinse. It helps re-establish the natural pH balance of your hair after shampooing, helps get rid of buildup caused by some shampoos and conditioners, and will make your hair glossy. Add one cup vinegar to three cups water or a strong infusion of rosemary, an herb beneficial for all hair types. Use about half as a rinse after shampooing. Add a drop of rosemary essential oil to your hairbrush before brushing and occasionally lower your head and brush from the back of the neck down to the ends—inversion gives your scalp a healthy rush of blood and increases circulation. Gently massaging the scalp is beneficial as well. Coat your fingertips in a light oil and use small circular motions all over the scalp with all ten fingertips. Any of these blends will be beneficial for facial hair as well.

For Dry Hair

If your hair is dry, lavender, rosemary, and ylang-ylang essential oils are beneficial. Try making a vinegar rinse with a marsh mallow or oatstraw infusion by adding two to three drops of either essential oil. You can also make a moisturizing oil by combining one tablespoon each jojoba and avocado oils and adding one drop each of lavender and ylang-ylang. Place in a cup or bottle in a bowl of hot water and allow it to get warm before using it after shampooing. Massage it gently into your scalp and then comb it through the rest of your hair. Leave it on for fifteen minutes to an hour and then rinse or wash out. Avoid washing your hair every day, as shampoo strips away the outer layer of oil that protects your hair. You may want to try combining equal parts ylang ylang and lavender and applying one drop of the mixture to your hairbrush each morning before you brush your hair.

For Oily Hair

For those who have oily hair, lemon, bergamot, geranium, and cypress are the essential oils to use. Make an oil treatment by using two tablespoons jojoba oil and adding one drop each of geranium and cypress. Jojoba is not actually an oil, but a wax, and is well known for its ability to normalize skin, whether it is oily or dry. You can also create a normalizing hair lotion by making an infusion of lavender and nettles. Put it in a spray bottle and lightly mist hair before brushing. You can add a beneficial essential oil if desired. People with oily hair should also avoid washing their hair every day. Washing too often can cause the oil glands in the scalp to work overtime to replace what was stripped off by the shampoo, making your hair even oilier. Protein-enhanced conditioners can also contribute to this condition. Use equal parts geranium and bergamot for a one-drop-daily hairbrush mixture for your hair type.

For Normal Hair

For those lucky few with normal hair make your oil treatment with sweet almond oil and rosemary or carrot essential oil. The normalizing lotion listed above will also help nourish and protect this type of hair. Rosemary is best for your hairbrush.

To refresh your hair color (and this works well whether or not your hair is dyed), try an herbal rinse. Take four tablespoons of your selected herb and steep it in two quarts of water (that has been brought to a boil and removed from heat) for twenty to twenty-five minutes. Strain and pour over hair repeatedly, using a bowl or sink to recycle the rinse. This treatment is best used just after washing hair. For blondes, chamomile is best; for brunettes, sage; for red heads, try calendula; and for gray hair, use rosemary. None of these herbs will really cause a drastic change in your hair color; they will help general health and shine. Sage or fresh walnut leaf used over a period of time will slightly darken hair. To lighten hair, make a rinse of one part fresh squeezed lemon juice to one part cider vinegar and take a walk in the sunlight.

Gels and Styling Products

If you ever use gel or mousse in your hair, try using aloe vera gel instead. It has an excellent hold, its moisturizing and astringent properties are very good for the scalp, and it washes out easily without leaving your hair dry or slightly sticky. Not only that, but you can add your favorite essential oils to make a hair gel with a pleasing, natural fragrance. Use about three drops of oil for every ounce of gel. The lighter, organic aloe vera gel can be used on dry hair without causing "helmet head." The stickiness that gels can sometimes leave you with is usually caused by an overabundance of holding agents that are doing more than your hair needs, leaving extra holding power available to attract dust and other particles that will dull your hair and weigh it down. Helmet head (where your hair actually feels hard and stiff after the gel has dried) is caused by the thickening agents that are once again overdoing it. These agents can also react to the alcohol in the products, making excess moisture evaporate out of the gel, leaving only the hard residue behind.

Shampoos and Conditioners

You can personalize your shampoo and conditioner by adding beneficial oils to them before you use them. Milder and fewer chemicals is preferable of course, but this is another very simple way to use essential oils for your hair. You can make your own shampoo using an infusion of soapwort or liquid castile soap with a little vinegar added. Of course, you can add essential oils to these, too! You can also make a conditioner using a very old recipe: Take an egg yolk and add it to two tablespoons of jojoba oil. Add one drop of rosemary essential oil and apply to clean hair. Leave on a few minutes and rinse with cool or lukewarm water. This will leave hair especially shiny.

If your scalp is dry and itchy, it may be dandruff, or, it may be a sensitivity to sodium laurel sulfate, a common ingredient in shampoos, which has come under fire at times as being highly irritating and even toxic. Research findings on this topic are contradictory; however, if you have a dry, itchy scalp you may want to try switching to a shampoo without this particular additive. You could also be experiencing a food-related allergy.

If you're sure your itchy scalp is due to dandruff, try adding a little tea tree, rosemary, or lavender essential oil to your regular shampoo instead of buying a dandruff shampoo, or try the following recipe: take four ounces of your regular shampoo (the less scent and chemicals, the better) and add five drops each of rosemary essential oil, thyme oil, and sage oil. Use evening primrose oil as a weekly conditioner. You may want to consider buying a tea tree shampoo from a health food store, which works well to keep dandruff manageable when used regularly.

When You Need Extra Strength

No one likes it when a child comes home from school with the dreaded note about lice. Instead of using expensive and toxic commercial shampoos (which effectively kill the parasites but are basically like putting pesticides on your head), you may want to try this natural remedy for lice: Take four tablespoons jojoba oil and add seven drops each of lavender and tea tree essential oil. Coat the scalp and hair well, wrap hair and scalp completely in plastic wrap and leave on for an hour or two. Carefully comb out hair to remove the (now dead) lice and nits. Repeat, if necessary, several days later. Thoroughly brushing at least twice a day will help prevent another infestation.

Organic Cosmetics

⫸ by Sally Cragin ⫷

Years ago as a geology major learning about minerals, I happened to look at my fabulous new eye shadow and noticed that the ingredients included micaceous ingredients (such as aluminum silicates) as well as talc.

Now, I really love minerals, but the idea of putting material that can be measured on Moh's Scale of Hardness on thin eyelid skin seemed a high price to pay for beauty. So I took note when a very creative company in western Massachusetts recently launched a new product line that puts a different spin on cosmetics ingredients. Suki (http://sukipure.com) offers a lip and cheek stain, tinted moisturizers, and liquid concealers that are entirely cream-based instead of powder-based.

While I've never had skin-care issues (still holding my breath with fingers crossed!), I have noticed over

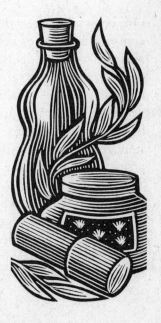

the years that most skin creams, oils, and moisturizers just don't feel right. This could be because of the parabens (chemicals made from petroleum) or some other polysyllabic substances that dominate the ingredients list of a shampoo bottle.

That's why I've always had an eye out for alternatives to mass-produced products. Fortunately, in my neighborhood, friends who keep bees have a small cottage industry manufacturing a skin cream out of beeswax, borax, distilled water, and mineral oil. You won't find Sulin Orchards Hand Cream beyond Fitchburg, Massachusetts, but chances are a home cosmetics cook is making their own version of this emollient, which I use for moisturizing dry winter skin. When my son was a baby, I used it as a diaper cream. (I've also used the cream as a chapstick).

Once you get into the habit of reading ingredients and learning a bit about some of the chemicals used by large manufacturers, it gets much easier to be an informed consumer or—given enough time, curiosity, and spare pots and pans—a home chemist.

Getting Started

Owner Suki Kramer, the founder of Suki Naturals started her company because of her own avowed fondness for "high-end personal-care products." Her product line is all natural, all organic, and vegan, and it uses some surprising ingredients, including shiitake (yes, the mushroom), burdock, green tea, and white willow. Agricultural historians will recall that white willow is one source of salicins, the main ingredient in aspirin. "We use standardized white willow," explains Kramer. "The analgesic properties help increase cell renewal."

Another woman-owned company in Massachusetts is Wiseways Herbals, which opened in 1987. Owner Miriam Massaro began her career as a "farmer/herb gatherer," a nature lover who experimented as an herbal healer for herself and friends, then started taking herbal products to expectant mothers. "We're nationwide now." Wiseways Herbals began a skin-care line for women a few years ago. The Oshuna skin-care line is named for the African River Goddess and uses natural olive, jojoba, grape seed, and other oils as a base with a variety of unusual and unexpected ingredients. The Camellia eye cream does indeed contain oil of Camellia, but also sea buckthorn (from Siberia), ashwaganda (Indian ginseng), and more familiar items such as aloe vera and comfrey.

"When I started there were very few (shops) out there, but the natural products industry is growing," says Massaro. "Maybe people are disillusioned with chemicals on their skin and in their bodies. I like to research the latest antioxidant longevity herbs, and take better care of myself."

Both companies manufacture their wares in small batches so that the product doesn't sit on a shelf. I've used a variety of products from both and enjoy the high quality—and reading the list of ingredients. For a part-time casual cosmetics cook, this is an education in itself.

Simple Skin-Care Recipes
(Exercise, Drink Water, Exercise)

The easiest improvement you can make in your skin-care regimen is to drink enough water. Dehydration comes more easily than you might think and if you are exercising regularly, you're moving liquids through your system more efficiently. I keep a pitcher with a filter on my desk and another bottle of unfiltered water so I don't always have to refill my pitcher. I drink water from a large glass because I've conditioned myself to empty the glass before leaving the desk, a lesson brought home after seeing my beloved little house cat sticking his head in the glass after I've gone!

I've always found it amusing to distinguish between face cream, body cream, and foot cream, but there is a difference. The parts of the body that get a more vigorous workout definitely need special attention.

Easy Foot Scrub

You can make a lovely scrub solution for foot calluses by adding a little cornmeal or powdered oatmeal (use a clean coffee grinder) to olive oil. Warm this up and, if you want an aromatherapy benefit, add a few drops of peppermint oil. Rinse with warm water.

Suki's Standby Recipe

When I asked Suki Kramer what products she used when she wasn't using her own, she reminded me of the best old standby: a honey/yogurt mask. Just a teaspoon of each mixed together and applied to the face can have a moisturizing and tightening effect. Rinse with warm water once it's dried, of course.

Struggling Artist Facial Steam

When I was starting out as a journalist, I was hesitant to try quality [expensive] products. Though enticing, essential oils were beyond my budget. One day I had a brainstorm after hearing about a friend warding off a cold with a facial steamer. Why not do a homemade version for pennies? All I used were rosemary leaves from the spice cabinet, a metal bowl, and a towel. Heat enough water to fill one-third of the bowl, add a couple of tablespoons of rosemary, cover your head with a towel, and breathe in as long as you can stand it. This is an easy way to work up a sweat and you don't have a facial steamer to take apart when you're done. You can also do this steam with essential oils. If your face needs extra moisturizing, try rose or chamomile. Oily skin could benefit from eucalyptus or lemon. Lavender oil works for normal or nontroubled skin.

Save-Your-Pipes Skin Scrubby

A lot of really interesting bath-oil recipes often have substances that could definitely clog your drain if you use them often enough. But you can make a bath scrubby in a muslin bag or just a square of cheesecloth if you use equal parts ground up oatmeal, dried orange peel, and pulverized almonds. You can also hang this little bag over your tap as you're filling the tub. Or do a variant with dried sage, thyme, or lavender.

Glycerin Soap Kits

Years ago, to do a story about a woman who made her own soap, I spent a morning with her while she concocted a very interesting brew on her stovetop. It took hours, and there was one thrilling and hazardous moment when she was handling a kettle of boiling lye. This adventure thoroughly convinced me that I wasn't cut out to be a soapmaker. If you're going to spend that much time stirring something on a blazing-hot stovetop, you might as well get brownies at the end of it.

Some time later, I noticed craft shops started selling glycerine to melt in the microwave and make your own soap. Since glycerine can dry your skin, I started experimenting with other substances to put in the soap bar to make it more skin-friendly. I never found a recipe that used honey and oatmeal that didn't smell rank, but tablespoons of really good olive oil would spark up a soap bar, as would ground-up cucumber. (Use this soap right away—even though the cucumber is part of the soap, it's still organic.) My most successful soap came from pulverizing some excellent lavender buds brought back from the south of France by fortunate relatives. I added a tablespoon per bar, and then a few drops of lavender oil when the soap wasn't red-hot anymore. The herbs added an astringent quality and a few drops of blue and red soap-coloring made for a handsome bar.

Interesting Homemade Toothpowder

When my cousin Susan Cragin and I went to Nebraska to visit the sites of her book, *Nuclear Nebraska*, she had forgotten her toothpaste and had to use a box of baking soda instead. That reminded me of variants of homemade tooth cleansers. You can dry a few tablespoons of sage leaves in the oven, crush them into powder, and add some kosher salt. You definitely want to rinse after using this, but the sage makes for an interesting taste in your mouth.

Hair Care

As we all know, hair is protein, and if you have weak nails or wispy hair (or a change in your hair due to trauma or sickness) consider helping your body recover by changing your eating habits. More vitamin C during a time of stress can be good for your locks. Citrus fruit and juice is an easy source of this, plus dark green vegetables and plants like broccoli and peppers. Protein sources include beans and peas; dairy products, including cheese, eggs, and milk; plus fish and meat. A few tablespoons of wheat germ in morning cereal can also give you extra protein.

You can make a dandruff rinse by boiling thyme with water—two tablespoons per cup of water. Let this material cool and strain out the plant matter before rubbing into clean, wet hair. Rinse this off after an hour and you should see an improvement in your scalp condition.

Dry Shampoo

Cornstarch really is a miracle ingredient. Essential in making homemade pudding, it's also a gentle powder when applied to baby's backside, and it's great to add to the innersoles of your shoes to deodorize. But did you know it's a great dry shampoo? Apply to dry hair, massage in and then brush out.

An Herbal Primer

When gathering herbs, avoid roadsides or areas where cars travel. The metals and chemicals in exhaust enter the soil, and the roots of nearby plants. It's best to gather herbs on private land, far from civilization, if possible.

Red Clover Blossoms

One folk remedy involving red clover blossoms can help alleviate skin inflammation, particularly insect bites. Mash or chop the flower and apply directly to skin. Some herbalists utilize the extract and it's being explored as a treatment for skin disorders, including psoriasis.

Purslane

Purslane grows around the world and virtually every culture has a use for it. Chances are, it grows in your yard as well. It's a low-growing weed with tiny oblate leaves growing parallel on a central stalk. Medicinal applications include serving as a balm for conditions ranging from stomach disorders, headache, and lack of milk flow in nursing mothers to skin disorders (smear the juice of the leaves on as a poultice). I like purslane because it's a handsome, subtle plant and you can always count on its return!

Aloe Vera

Aloe is an amazingly durable plant and highly forgiving. Give it a sunny windowsill and an occasional drink of water and it will joyously grow spiked leaves in a hurry. The first time I saw aloe used for sunburn was in Jamaica. Folks were selling long spears of the leaf to all the Europeans who were getting lobster-red after their first day on the sand. But you don't need a big plant to have enough for home use. To use the gel, snip off an inch of leaf, squeeze out the juice and apply to skin for sunburn or other inflammation. I've also read that aloe vera gel and juice can be helpful for oral health, but haven't tried this myself.

Fennel

Fennel looks much like a large version of its relative, dill. Like dill, this herb has a score of herbal remedy and culinary uses. You could grind up roasted seeds and add it to the "Interesting Homemade Toothpowder" recipe. You could also chew it for a breath refresher and it's a helpful digestive aid (specifically, a "carminative" so it's capable of diminishing gas). No, I haven't found specific cosmetic uses for it, but I love the taste!

Lemon

Though not an herb, lemon is an all-purpose ingredient for a skin toner. Early California surfers knew that if you put a lot of lemon juice in your hair, you'd get a sun-streaked look after a day on the sand (current parlance: "layin' out" according to a surfer-chick cousin). And a quickie skin-toner can be made by making a cup of peppermint tea, letting it cool, and adding about a tablespoon of lemon juice. Add a couple of tablespoons of witch hazel if you like, and daub on with a cotton ball. You can refrigerate the rest for up to a week or so. (We need someone to invent a very small refrigerator to go in the bathroom. Many homemade cosmetics need to be chilled to prevent decay.)

Easy Sugar Scrub

When did the sugar scrub become a "spa" treatment? The grains of sugar are an exfollient and mixed with oil, can make your skin feel wonderful. I did a lot of investigating before realizing it was easier to expand on a sample batch than to make a lot of this all at once. The basic recipe is simple: one part oil, two parts sugar.

Mix two tablespoons of sugar and one tablespoon of oil (grapeseed, jojoba, or almond preferably, but using olive oil isn't as dire as you may think. Walnut oil is too fragrant and can make you feel like a salad bowl). You want the sugar to be saturated, but not swimming in the oil. Add essential oils as a flavoring (or just some lemon juice to sharpen the aroma). Grapefruit essential oil is the most frequently used in a sugar scrub, but lavender or calendula is pleasant. Scrub on a damp face, massage, and rinse well. Keep in a dark place and don't make too much at a time. (The maximum seems to be one cup of sugar and a half cup of oil.)

On Making Cosmetics for Gifts

Always use very small jars that have been sanitized (boiling usually does the trick). Because these products contain no preservatives, advise your giftee to use it as soon as possible. The biggest expense in making a collection of sugar scrubs or skin scrubbies are the containers (amber jars and muslin bags). This is where creative recycling can be useful. You can also make the skin scrubbies out of a double-layer of cheesecloth.

Flower Power Beauty Parlor

≈ by Zaeda Yin ≈

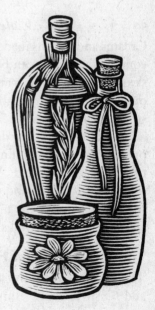

Fragrant flowers, herbs, and fruit have long been used in beauty treatments to refresh, cleanse, soothe, and enhance the complexion. Natural homemade preparations cost a fraction of expensive cosmetics found in department stores, health care shops, and pharmacies that contain chemicals and preservatives. More often than not, we pay more for the fancy packaging of commercial products than the product itself! Although homemade beauty products do not contain preservatives and will not keep forever, commercial beauty products also have a shelf life between one and three years, depending on the preservatives used.

Beauty products made at home are as effective (if not more potent) as commercial ones. Making them yourself gives the satisfaction of your own personal touch, creativity, and innovative ideas. Recipes are quick, easy, delicate, harmless, inexpensive, and additive-free. They can be made for personal use or given as gifts to family and friends. Matching sets can be made to suit individual needs. If you give any natural homemade beauty products as presents, be sure to take into account the intended recipient's skin type and any allergies that they may have.

Before rolling up your sleeves and getting started, collect a variety of pretty and unusual jars, bottles, and other glass containers in different shapes, colors, and sizes with lids, screw-tops, glass-stoppers, and corks. Wash and sterilize them. After drying, store them in a cupboard for future use as you traverse along merry ways of producing your own natural beauty preparations. Always remember to keep natural beauty-care items in a cool place, preferably away from sunlight. Some can be stored in the refrigerator until ready for use. The following simple recipes contain easily obtainable ingredients for making beauty products that pamper from face to foot.

Violet Cream Cleanser

Creams and lotions made with violets will help to improve a dull complexion. They can be used morning or night to cleanse the skin, leaving it smooth and soft. You will need 1 ounce lanolin, 1 ounce cocoa butter, 4 tablespoons almond oil, and 4 tablespoons strong violet infusion.

Melt the lanolin and cocoa butter together in a bowl placed over a saucepan of boiling water. Stir occasionally until the mixture is evenly blended. Add almond oil and stir again. Remove the bowl from heat and whisk in the violet infusion. When it is slightly cool, pour the mixture into a clean, sterilized screw-top jar. Give the jar a good shake before using.

Floral Facial Cleansing Soap

This simple soap is suitable for all skin types, including delicate and sensitive skins. You will need 10 tablespoons finely grated castille soap, 8 tablespoons boiling water, 2 tablespoons crushed dried flowers of chamomile, lavender, jasmine, and rose petals; and 4 drops sandalwood essential oil.

Melt the castille soap with water in a bowl placed over a saucepan of boiling water. Stir frequently until the mixture becomes smooth. Crush the dried flowers to a fine powder. Remove the bowl of castille soap from the saucepan. Stir in the powdered flowers with sandalwood essential oil. Mix thoroughly. Pour into a bottle and label.

Rose Petal Facial Mask

Another thorough facial cleansing method is a facial mask or "face pack" prior to applying toner and moisturizer. Making a good face pack involves mixing a strong flower or herbal infusion with a thickening agent to form a paste. An easy method for the beginner is to pour ½ cup of boiling water onto 1 to 2 handfuls of rose petals in a heatproof container to make the infusion. Leave the rose petals to infuse for 15 to 30 minutes. Strain and let the liquid cool. Oatmeal or yogurt can be added to the infusion to thicken the face pack. For a full-bodied, thick facial mask, rose petals can be added directly to oatmeal or yogurt and left to permeate for at least 30 minutes before spreading over a clean face, avoiding the eyes and mouth. Lie back and relax until the face pack dries. Wash with warm water and finish by splashing with cold water.

Tonic for Oily Skin

Oily skins can benefit from the gentleness of this toning tonic, which removes the last traces of makeup, dead cells, dirt, cleanser, or soap from the face. You will need 2 fluid ounces witch hazel, 2 fluid ounces rose water, and 1 fluid ounce orange flower water.

Simply blend the ingredients together and pour into a bottle with a glass-stopper or screw-cap.

Lime Flower Toner

Lime flower toner is useful for removing impurities and as an astringent for tightening skin pores. You will need 1 ounce dried lime flowers and 4 ounces boiling water.

Boil the lime flowers in a saucepan for 15 to 25 minutes then leave to cool slightly. Strain off the liquid, firmly pressing the flowers down. Pour into a thick glass bottle and let it cool to room temperature before sealing and labeling.

Angelica Ointment for Itchy Skin

For soothing itchy skin, an angelica ointment made from fresh leaves and a tiny sprinkling of 2 crushed angelica flowers can provide tremendous relief. Melt a small jar of petroleum jelly slowly in the top part of a double-boiler. Add a handful of finely crushed angelica leaves and a bit of the crushed flowers. Stir well using a stainless steel or wooden spoon. Leave the mixture to slowly infuse for an hour. Strain into small glass pots and let them cool down. Secure the pots with lids when the ointment is cold.

Borage Lotion for Ridding Spots

Borage flowers dry well and also retain their lovely colors. They help to clear the skin of troublesome spots when combined with dandelion and watercress. A simple method is to blend and mix equal quantities of borage, dandelion, and watercress into a juice for use as a lotion. Wash the face and towel dry. Gently spread the lotion over affected parts, but avoid the eyes. Allow the lotion to dry completely and wash the face again. Always prepare a fresh mixture for each application. With patience and repeated use of this recipe, blemishes and pimples will diminish.

Cornflower Moisturizer

Cornflower beauty preparations are suitable for all skin types. After making the moisturizer below, apply to the skin using your fingertips. Work upwards from the jaw to the eyes and then across the forehead. You will need 2 tablespoons lanolin, 3 tablespoons almond oil, 3 tablespoons beeswax, 3 tablespoons thick natural honey, and 3 tablespoons strong cornflower infusion (i.e. 2 table-spoons fresh flowers to ¼ pint spring water).

Place the lanolin, almond oil, beeswax, and honey in a bowl placed over a saucepan of boiling water. Let the contents melt gradually and gently stir until evenly blended. Add the cornflower infusion and stir for another 2 minutes. Remove from heat and continue stirring until the moisturizer becomes smooth, creamy, thick, and cold. Spoon into an attractive glass jar or pot, seal, and label.

Fennel or Chamomile Eye Care

Sore or inflamed eyes will benefit from a soothing eye-bath infusion of restorative herbs such as chamomile or fennel. Pour the infusion into a plastic eye bath (cup bought from the pharmacy). Cup the eye bath to the eye, tilt the head back and blink a few times, gently allowing the infusion to "swish" around the eyeball. Repeat this procedure whenever required. Strong infusions of chamomile or fennel tea can be utilized for eye compresses by dipping 2 pieces of soft lint gauze into the infusion and placing over closed eyes for a minimum of 15 minutes.

Herbal Eye Gel

A simple homemade eye gel is toning and rejuvenates delicate skin around the eyes. This herbal recipe uses a decoction of dried chamomile, calendula, and marsh mallow leaves. In a saucepan, place 1 tablespoon of each herb in 25 ounces of cold water. Bring the mixture to a boil. Reduce heat and let it simmer until the liquid is reduced to ¼ of the original volume. Wash the saucepan and heat 12 tablespoons of the decoction with 4 tablespoons of double-distilled witch hazel until it reaches just below boiling point. Add ½ teaspoon of agar and stir until the mixture is well-blended or dissolved. ("Agar" or "agar-agar" are seaweeds, especially *Gracilaria lichenoides* from which a gelatinous substance is extracted for use as a solidifying or jelling agent.) Pour the eye gel into a jar and let it cool before sealing and labeling. Apply to the eyes in the morning after cleansing the face and before bedtime.

Calendula Lip Balm

Regular use of a lip balm will soothe and prevent dry, cracked, or chapped lips in all weather conditions. Calendula-based balm keeps well in most temperatures except extremely hot and humid weather, when refrigeration may be required. Prepare a cup of calendula oil by placing 4 tablespoons of fresh calendula petals in a glass jar. Drizzle 1 cup of cold-pressed almond oil over the petals. Cover tightly and place the jar on a windowsill that catches daily sunlight. Leave the jar there for 5 days in summer and 7 to 15 days during winter. Traditionally in folk preparations, this method is called "sunlight infusion." Strain by pressing firmly to extract all the oil from the petals.

Prepare the lip balm by putting the calendula oil in the top portion of a double saucepan while the bottom part bubbles with boiling water. Add 1 teaspoon each of beeswax, natural honey, and wheat-germ oil. Constantly stir the contents. When the mixture becomes smooth, pour the hot solution into a wide-mouth ointment jar. Leave to cool then seal tightly. Wait until the lip balm is hardened before applying to the lips.

Rose Geranium and Lavender Massage Oil

This is one of the most soothing massage oils to use after a long day of stress or physical exhaustion. It eases tension and relaxes the body and mind, bringing a sense of relaxation and well-being. This recipe makes about 1 cup. You will need ¼ cup rose geranium petals, ¼ cup lavender flowers, and 1 cup apricot oil

Place petals in a glass jar. Gently warm the apricot oil in a saucepan on very low heat. Pour over petals and seal. Leave in a warm place for two weeks, shaking the jar at least twice a day. After two weeks, pour the jar's contents into the saucepan and warm slightly on low heat. Strain through muslin or cheesecloth, discard the flower petals. Pour the oil into bottles and seal. For a more pungent fragrance, repeat the process using fresh petals.

Flax-Linseed and Bergamot Bath Oil

Linseed from the flax plant and its flowers are effective for softening the skin. It also makes a soothing, relaxing bath—just put a handful of flax and linseed into a muslin cloth bag, tie it, and add to bath water. To make a bath oil containing these ingredients, combine into a bowl 1 cup of fresh flax flowers and linseed, ¼ cup cold-pressed olive oil, ½ cup pure alcohol, ¼ cup rose water, and ¼ cup distilled water. Cover and steep for 2 days. Strain and then add 1 teaspoon of bergamot essential oil. Blend the mixture thoroughly. Insert a fresh sprig of flower into an attractive glass bottle and carefully pour the mixture into it. Seal and label.

Avocado and Lavender Body Cream

Body creams are applied after showers or baths to moisturize body skin. They can also be massaged on hands, arms, thighs, legs, and feet. The following recipe is rich, nourishing, and suitable for all skin types. You will need 2 teaspoons beeswax, 3 fluid ounces avocado oil, 1 teaspoon lavender essential oil, 2 tablespoons rosewater, and a pinch of borax.

Pour some water into the bottom part of a double-boiler and set it on low to medium heat. Put beeswax, avocado oil, and lavender essential oil in the top part of the double boiler. Let the contents heat gently. Stir regularly with a wooden spoon until the beeswax melts and the entire mixture is smooth. Blend the rose water into the borax. Remove the top part of the double boiler from heat and blend the rose water and borax mix into the boiler's contents. Keep stirring until the cream is cool and smooth. Pour into sterilized jars, seal, and label.

Marigold Hand Cream

Make a strong infusion of marigold petals by pouring ½ cup of boiling water over 1 tablespoon of petals and letting it cool down completely. Strain the liquid into a small saucepan and mix it with 2 teaspoons of glycerin and 2 teaspoons of arrowroot powder. Stir the mixture over low heat until it becomes thick and creamy. Remove from heat and add 5 drops each of lavender and lemon balm essential oils. Thoroughly mix the contents and wait till the cream is slightly cool before pouring into a wide-mouthed jar with a screw-top lid. When the cream reaches room temperature, put the lid on. Label the jar and store in a cool place. If intending to give as a present, cut a piece of pretty lace to fit over the lid and tie a ribbon around it.

Rosemary Foot Bath

For swollen, tired, and sweaty feet, a rosemary foot bath used at least twice a week will help reduce excessive perspiration and keep bacteria at bay. Make an infusion of rosemary with a cup of boiling water poured onto a handful of rosemary in a bowl and set aside for 25 minutes. Strain the infusion and add to a basin of lukewarm water. Soak the feet for at least 15 minutes. More warm water can be added to the basin if desired, especially if you intend to soak the feet a little longer.

Honeysuckle Foot Balm

The feet need as much pampering as other parts of the body. Foot balms are soothing to tired feet and help prevent dry skin. The recipe below makes about ½ cup. You will need ⅓ cup lanolin, 3 tablespoons almond oil, 3 tablespoons glycerine, and ¼ teaspoon honeysuckle oil.

Place lanolin, almond oil, and glycerin in the top part of a double saucepan over simmering water. Stir until the mixture is smoothly combined with even texture. Add honeysuckle oil and stir contents for another minute. Remove from heat. Patiently continue stirring until the mixture is completely cool. Pour into small jars, seal, and label.

Lovely Lavender

❧ by Danny Pharr ❧

Tiny violet flowers arranged in pipe-cleaner fashion and displayed at the end of musty green stalks sparsely covered with thin, pointed leaves is the hallmark image of lavender. However, lavender is best remembered for its most fragrant scent. The smell of lavender sprigs in linen closets and dresser drawers triggers memories of childhood, a freshly made bed, cookies, and that one corner of the garden where just brushing by the lavender released its fragrance.

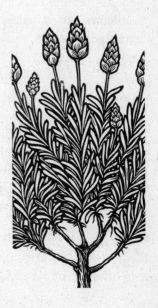

Lavender was long used by the Romans to scent their oft-indulged recreational baths, although lavender was not scientifically classified until the eighteenth century, some 1,700 years later. Swedish naturalist Carolus Linnaeus classified the genus of lavender, using the Latin word *lavandus*, which means "to wash." European lavender was given the species name, *stoechas*, which applied to all plants of a pale gray color. The main lavender varieties are Spanish, French, and English, though subvarieties abound.

Lavender grows best in full sun and prefers well-drained, light, airy, soil. The plant is susceptible to fungus, but good air circulation will help deter or prevent the disease. Root rot is also a concern in wet climates, so fast-draining soil will also help.

Harvest lavender only on cool, sunny mornings after the dew has evaporated, and even then, only after a string of two or three sunny days. Harvesting lavender after dry weather shortens the drying process. The cool morning air allows the lavender oil to remain collected in the flower buds.

Drying lavender is best done in dark, dry, areas of well-circulated air. During the hot summer months, lavender will dry in a week or two. The flowers can be laid on newspaper or bundled and hung to dry. Check for mold every couple of days.

Lavender has been so coveted for its wonderfully refreshing scent that people have spent the last two thousand years inventing new ways to capture its essence. Most often used for scenting bed clothes and chests of drawers, lavender is an ingredient in medicines, soaps, baked goods, body lotions, incense, alcoholic beverages, massage oils, cooking spices, and crafts.

Culinary Uses

Spring in France is marked by the annual Parisian pilgrimage to lavender fields of Provence where they pick lavender buds and leaves for the season's dining delights. Cooking with lavender is an adventure into the culinary arts. Use it as a spice or mix it with salt or sugar to give any dish a hint of lavender. Substitute lavender for sage or rosemary, as they are all from the sage (Salvia) family. Try some of these recipes.

Delicious Iced Lavender Cookies

Begin by preheating an oven to 375 degrees F. and creaming 1 cup of sugar into ½ cup of butter. To the butter and sugar, add 2 teaspoons of dried and crushed food-grade lavender flower buds, 1½ cups flour, 2 teaspoons baking powder, and a double pinch of kosher salt. Bind this rather dry mixture with 3 lightly beaten eggs. Once you have achieved a fairly consistent dough, drop spoonfuls of dough onto an ungreased cookie sheet. Give the dough about 2 inches clearance to allow for spreading. Smaller cookies will bake better. While the cookies bake for about 12 minutes (being careful to watch closely for the last 3 minutes to avoid overbaking), make the icing by combining 1 tablespoon and 1 teaspoon of rose water, 1 tablespoon of tap water, and 1½ cups of powdered sugar. Stir this mixture until the sugar is dissolved and the icing is smooth. Once the cookies have cooled sufficiently, drizzle the icing in lines over the cookies and enjoy.

Lavender Salt

In a spice grinder, mix 1 tablespoon of dried and crushed food-grade lavender flower buds and a double pinch of coarse kosher salt. For larger quantities, use 1½ teaspoons of salt for every cup of lavender buds. Adjust the salt content to your taste.

Lavender Sugar

Mix 1 cup of superfine sugar with 1 tablespoon of dried and crushed food-grade lavender flower buds in a food processor. Grind the mixture until the lavender buds have become powder and the mixture is a consistent color and texture.

Lavender Herb de Provence

Hand mix equal amounts of dried and crushed food-grade lavender flower buds, dried basil, dried rosemary, dried thyme, dried savory, and dried marjoram. Adjust the quantities to your taste and use to enhance the flavors of beef, chicken, pork, lamb, rabbit, soups, sauces, and vegetables.

Lavender Butter

Soften one stick of unsalted butter. In a mixing bowl, cream together the softened butter, 1 tablespoon of dried and crushed food-grade lavender flower buds, ¼ teaspoon coarse kosher salt, and ¼ teaspoon finely grated lemon zest. Using the top of a butter serving dish lined on the inside with wax paper and then plastic wrap to create a trough, spoon the creamed butter into the trough, smooth the surface, and chill back to stick form. Remove the wax paper trough wrapping from the butter server, remove the wax paper and plastic from the butter, and serve the stick of lavender butter as desired.

Grilled Lavender Rack of Lamb

Set the rack of lamb on the counter under a kitchen towel and allow the rack to come to room temperature. Rub the rack on all surfaces with lavender salt and allow the rack to sit another 30 minutes. Meanwhile, start the grill for a medium heat. Grill the rack of lamb on all sides until golden and juicy.

Honey Lavender Ice Cream

Bring to a slight boil, 2 cups of heavy cream, 1 cup half-and-half, ¼ cup dried and crushed food-grade lavender flower buds, and ½ cup clover honey, stirring occasionally. Let the cream mixture steep for 20 minutes. Strain the cream mixture to remove the lavender buds and return to the cleaned saucepan over medium heat until hot but not boiling. Meanwhile, blend together 6 egg yolks, ¼ cup raw sugar, and ⅛ teaspoon of kosher salt. Whisk 1 cup of the cream mixture into the egg yolks until well blended, then add the egg and cream mixture back to the pot of hot cream. Cook over low heat until the hot custard will coat the back of a wooden spoon. Pour the custard into a bowl and cool completely by placing the bowl in an ice-water bath in a larger bowl. Freeze the custard in an ice cream maker.

Roasted Lavender Cornish Hens

Preheat oven to 475 degrees F. Wash the hens, discard the gizzards, and pat dry. Push a slice of butter and a few fresh thyme leaves under the skin of each thigh and both sides of the breast.

Tie the legs with kitchen string and secure the wings with wooden toothpicks. Rub the hen with fresh-squeezed lemon juice and place in a roasting pan. Roast the bird in the middle of the oven for about 45 minutes, basting occasionally. When the juices run clear and skin is golden brown, transfer the hen to a warmed plate. Add ¼ cup of dessert wine, such as Sauternes, and deglaze the roasting pan over medium heat. Transfer *jus* to a saucepan and reduce to ¼ or ½ cup, serving from one to four hens.

Lavender Mashed Potatoes

When making mashed potatoes, the general rule is one russet per person plus one—five potatoes to serve four. Peel, chop, and boil 5 russets with kosher salt until the potato chunks can be smashed with the flat of a fork. Simmer 1 cup of half-and-half with 1 tablespoon dried and crushed food-grade lavender flower buds. Soften ½ stick of butter. Strain the potatoes and place in a mixing bowl with the butter, then mash. Add the lavender-infused cream slowly while whipping the potatoes. Season with kosher salt and pepper.

Living with Lavender

Lavender can also be used around the home to freshen clothes, bed sheets, towels, scent the air, and to relax after a long day. Try some of these ideas.

Lavender Bath Sachet

Either purchase or sew a 3 × 2-inch muslin bag. Any size will work, but larger bags are not needed. If sewing a bag, cut a piece of muslin about 3½ × 4½ inches. Fold the muslin in half along the short axis creating a 3½ × 2¼-inch bag. Sew one long seam and a shorter seam. Turn the bag inside out and stuff with lavender buds. Turn the unfinished edges of the bag opening inside and sew the bag closed. This sachet should be used like a tea bag for a hot bath. Toss it in as the tub fills with water. Lavender can be tossed directly into the tub, but it will be a little messy to clean.

Lavender Linen Spray

Place 1 teaspoon, or about 100 drops, of lavender essential oil in a large spray bottle along with 2 ounces of formulator's alcohol, and shake well. Add 24 ounces of distilled water and shake again. The mixture will cloud immediately and separate over time. Shake well before each use. Spray on linens to freshen and scent.

Lavender Scented Sachet

Making a scented sachet is similar to making a bath sachet except that a prettier fabric should be used and some other ingredients should be added. Silk or satin, maybe organza, will make a nice initial presentation, and the addition of rose petals, potpourri, and a few drops of essential oils will create a wonderful and complex scent. Start by cutting a 10 × 5-inch piece from your chosen fabric. Fold the fabric in half along the short axis with the right side turned inside. Sew the bag along two sides. Mix the flowers in equal amounts and add a couple of drops of fragrant essential oil to the mix. Turn the bag inside out, right side out, stuff the bag, fold the unfinished edges in, and sew the bag closed. To present as a gift, make three sachets and tie them together with a wide ribbon and decorate with dried flowers or beads. Place the scented sachet in linen drawers, with the unmentionables, or any place a fresh lavender scent would be appreciated.

Multiple Uses, Many Methods

Lavender has long been thought to discourage depression, relieve headaches, insomnia, and stress. A lavender bath is one method for taking advantage of the calming fragrance. Sleeping with a dream pillow of lavender under the regular pillow will promote sweet gentle dreams. Relaxing with a lavender eye pillow laid across the eyes and temples will help to relieve the stress of overworked eyes, a common occurrence in these days of computer screens, television, and ever-smaller type.

Cosmetics of Ancient Egypt—Today!

⤳ by Sorita d'Este ⤳

The image of Cleopatra as a beautiful and desirable woman is one of the most enduring of the ancient world. Famed for her beauty and her ability to use it (illustrated by her beguiling of powerful men, including Julius Caesar and Mark Antony!) part of her reputation was undoubtedly founded on her use of cosmetics. The Egyptians were considered pioneers of this field. Four thousand years ago in ancient Egypt, beauty shops thrived by utilizing treatments that could still rival the best being offered by modern beauticians today. Treatments that originated in ancient Egyptian beauty shops include antiwrinkle treatments, hair extensions, facials, hair-removal, and makeup, as well as rejuvenating facials. Indeed, Cleopatra was said to have written a book on beauty secrets. Many of today's popular cosmetics

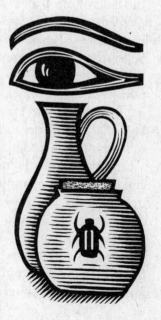

were just as renowned in ancient Egypt. These include black eyeliner (kohl), colored "green" eye shadows, "malachite" lip gloss, rouge, and even nail paints.

This clearly illustrates that the concerns we hold about our appearance today are not just a product of the modern world.

The desert environment of Egypt prompted its residents to make regular bathing an essential part of their lifestyle, along with the regular application of perfumes, deodorants, and cosmetics. Typical Egyptians would wash upon awaking, and again before and after their main meals. Wealthier households often had foot baths by the main doorways to their homes so visitors could wash off the dirt from the street before entering.

Though they had the same purpose, these early deodorants were extremely messy compared to the sprays or roll-ons we know today. They were made by mixing scented herbs, barks, resins, and perfumed oils with porridge. This mixture was then rolled into balls and placed in the armpits and between the legs. Those unable to afford the expensive perfumes and oils would rub balls of carob all over themselves to overcome body odors.

Although no recipes for soap had yet been discovered, we know that the Egyptians were very fond of their cleansing creams. Several of the medical *papyri* give a recipe for a body scrub used by ladies of the court. This scrub was made by mixing equal parts of powdered calcite (lime), salt, honey, and red natron, then grinding it all together to make a paste, which would be applied to the body daily. Natron is a purifying preservative that is still available today, though in declining use. The ancient Egyptians used it for a variety of purposes including mummification, mouthwashes, and other cleansing ointments. Red natron contains particles of iron, coloring the usual creamy white substance red. A slightly different recipe on record for this body scrub simply omits the powdered calcite.

Creams and oils were considered such an important aid in preventing the skin from cracking in the dry desert heat that they formed part of the wages for builders of the pyramids. Records indicate instances in which the workers would complain and protest vigorously when they did not receive their oils—sometimes to the point of lodging formal complaints.

Every Egyptian man and woman, from the lowest peasant to the Pharaoh, took great care of their appearance. Everyone owned a razor for removing body hair or used depilating scrubs for the same purpose. Great care was taken of hair, with shampoo, hair-coloring, and baldness remedies being widely used. However, not all these ancient unguents were as pleasant as our romantic ideas of ancient Egypt may suggest. For example, the hair-removing scrubs had some ingredients that would make most modern women squirm—like fly dung and ground up bird bones. Hair removal in ancient Egypt suddenly seems a great deal less pleasant!

Luckily not all the ingredients they used were quite as gruesome! Indeed many of the ingredients frequently used in cosmetics by the ancient Egyptians will be familiar to users of aromatherapy oils and incenses today. Popular ingredients included frankincense, myrrh, galbanum, lotus, lily, and sweet flag (calamus). Likewise, the base oils they used that are still in use today include almond, castor oil, linseed, olive, safflower, and sesame. Honey and wine were also often used as perfume bases.

A Little Mascara? (The Eyes Have It!)

For the creation of eye paints, minerals were pounded into fine powder and added to fats, oils, or honey. Malachite stones were used to create a bright green, lapis lazuli for blue, and galena for black. The color red represented chaos and danger to the Egyptians, while also symbolizing power and magic. To create red for use in lip glosses, nail paints, and rouge, the herb henna and red ochre were used as colorings, then mixed with fats and applied to the skin with a brush or spatula.

Today we know that galena (lead sulphide) should not be applied to the skin because over time can result in lead-poisoning. However, most Egyptians never reached their fortieth birthday, so lead toxicity was not a looming consideration. If you decide to follow old recipes for kohl containing lead sulphate, substitute it with a harmless ingredient like soot, which was also used in later Egypt for its blackening quality.

The Egyptians used eye makeup for more than its beauty enhancing qualities; it was also used to provide protection. The Egyptian word for "makeup palette" comes from the root "to protect" and eye makeup was thought to protect the wearer from the evil eye. By applying it around the eyes you prevented someone from fixing the evil eye on you!

Scents and Perfumes

The Egyptians loved their perfumes, and the best known of these was "Susinum," or "Oil of Lilies." Lily flowers were one of the most popular of all scents. Women probably viewed this oil as the Chanel of its day! The process of making the oil was laborious and complex, but the end result was considered well worthwhile. The recipe for making Oil of Lilies is included below—I have reduced the proportions down from the original recipe as it was always made in bulk!

Recipe for Oil of Lilies

Items: 100 lilies, 12½ ounces sweet almond oil, 4 ounces sweet flag, 4 teaspoons myrrh, ¾ teaspoon crocus, 1 tablespoon cinnamon, 1¾ ounces red wine, ⅓ cup cardamom, sea salt, rainwater.

1. Mix 7 ounces almond oil, 4 ounces sweet flag, and ¾ teaspoon myrrh in 1¾ ounces of red wine. Boil this mixture, and then strain.

2. Bruise and soak ⅓ cup cardamom in rainwater (or distilled water), and add this to the strained oil. Leave the mixture to soak and then strain.

3. Take 50 lilies, strip off all their leaves and place them in a broad, shallow vessel. Pour ⅓ cup of the oil over them, anoint your hands with honey, and stir the pot with your hands. Leave the mixture for 24 hours.

4. Strain off the oil, pouring it into another vessel lined with honey, and sprinkle a little salt onto it. Remove any impurities from the surface as they gather.

5. Take the remaining herbs, add another ⅓ cup of oil and ⅜ teaspoon crushed cardamom; stir and strain. Sprinkle with salt and set them aside. Repeat this process to make a third batch.

6. Take another 50 lilies, strip them as before, and repeat stages 3 to 5 with them.

7. Take ½ tablespoon myrrh, ⅜ teaspoon crocus, and 2 teaspoons cinnamon, beat them all, sift, and add to water.

8. Pour on the first batch of oil, skim the oil off after mixing, and store in small pots.

9. Repeat stage 7 for the other two batches of oil.

Greek writers including Pliny and Dioscorides wrote about the skill of the Egyptian perfumers, and Theophrastus went into some detail in his work *Concerning Odours*. One perfume sold throughout the Mediterranean was called "The Egyptian," and was made from myrrh and cinnamon steeped in oil. This perfume was also known as the "Mendesian," after the city of Mendes where it was made. Egyptian perfumes were often named after the city of their origin and manufacture.

Recipe for The Egyptian

Items needed: 9 ounces balanos oil, 16 ounces myrrh, ½ tablespoon cinnamon.

Add the 16 ounces myrrh resin to the 9 ounces of oil. (As balanos oil is very difficult to obtain, you can use sweet almond oil instead.) Allow to steep for a month. Add the cinnamon and allow to steep for another month. Strain and use the oil.

Other famous perfumes purportedly named after places include Stakte, which was made from myrrh added to balanos oil, and Cyprinum, which was also named after a plant now believed to be henna. Cyprinum was mixed with cardamom, cinnamon, myrrh, and southernwood.

Enduring and Endearing Qualities

Egyptian perfumes were made to exacting standards and expected to have a long shelf life. One bottle of Susinum would smell just like another; this quality control was one reason for the Egyptian supremacy in the ancient world of perfumery and cosmetics.

Not only did the Egyptians make the best cosmetics, but they also packaged them attractively. Pretty bottles are not a modern invention, as the Egyptians used delicate perfume jars made of alabaster, which was believed to ensure perfumes kept their scent longer. These jars have been found in archaeological digs dating back to the very first Egyptian dynasty—possibly even earlier. The name of the Egyptian cat-goddess Bastet is derived from these jars, which were called bas jars, as it translates as "She of the bas jar."

It was not only the women who wore perfume in ancient Egypt. Cyprinum was well known as a male perfume, perhaps because it had a lighter scent, or because it was easier to make and had fewer ingredients. It was made by boiling henna seeds in olive oil, then crushing the seeds and leaving it to soak. The oil was then strained and sold as a perfume.

Apart from perfumes and porridge balls, the Egyptians had another way of smelling fragrant that may seem rather bizarre today. Solid fat cones were perfumed and fixed to the head on top of the wig. As they melted, the wig would absorb the fat and become more fragrant with the scents. It did, of course, mean that you might have fat running down your face at times when you were eating or entertaining!

The most popular scents used in perfumes amongst the ancient Egyptians were:

Cedar (*Cedrus libani A. Rich.*): With its rich earthy scent, cedar was universally popular to wear and burn.

Cinnamon (*Cinnamomum zeylanicum Breyn*): The spicy, warm fragrance was very popular for its smell and also had beneficial antibacterial qualities.

Frankincense (*Boswellia carterii Birdw*): Considered the most holy of smells, this uplifting, clean citrus-like smell was imported in great quantity.

Labdanum (*Cistus creticus L*): Derived from the rockrose shrub, this sweet smell was very popular as an ingredient in perfumes because it brought out other sweet smells.

Lily (*Latin term*): One of the most popular scents for women for its distinctively strong, somewhat spicy qualities.

Mastic (*Pistacia lenticus L*): The gentle scent of mastic was a popular perfume thought to be pleasing to the gods.

Myrrh (*Commiphora myrrha Nees*): The earthy, stimulating scent was considered sensual and symbolic of female eroticism, and was also imported in quantity.

Sandalwood (*Santala album*): Imported from India, this scent was popular among the rich for its warm and sensual fragrance.

Storax (*Liquidambar styraciflua L.*): The calming and sensual scent of storax was very popular in perfumes for seduction.

Of course, the use of plants in cosmetics has never been limited to producing perfumes. Other cosmetic plants include:

Aloe Vera (*Aloe vera L.*): Widely used as an external salve for burns and skin problems, aloe vera was also taken internally for worms and ulcers. Aloe vera was added to wine and ground baked cucumber to make an ointment for treating skin disease.

Fenugreek (*Trigonella foenum-graecum L.*): This was used in an ointment to make people look younger and remove wrinkles, a very poplar treatment even then. Fenugreek added to honey was used for respiratory disorders and to reduce swellings.

Henna (*Lawsonia inermis L.*): Often used for its red dye, henna flowers also have a sweet fragrance used in perfumes.

Red ochre and **kohl** ground together and mixed with sycamore juice was used as a treatment for burn scars, and frankincense in honey was used for the same purpose.

A popular and allegedly successful wrinkle remedy was made of equal parts of cyperus grass, frankincense resin, fresh moringa oil, and wax, all ground finely and mixed with fermented plant juice and then applied daily. Even facial wraps have their origins in ancient Egypt, including the documented use of a carob and honey bandage as an antiwrinkle treatment among women.

Egyptian Foresight

The Egyptians knew that the eyes are the door to the soul and used a range of cosmetics to make their eyes more noticeable. One Egyptian love poem has the girl say the words "Like eye paint is my desire. When I see you, it makes my eyes sparkle," showing their awareness of such artifice. Eye paints made from ground malachite (green) or lapis lazuli (blue) or galena (black) were applied with a moistened stick from vases or tubes in which they were stored after being mixed. The minerals were kept in small linen or leather bags and ground on a palette to a fine powder when needed.

Eyewashes and cosmetics for cooling the eyes were also used. A simple eyewash was made from ground celery and hemp in pure water. Eye-cooling mixtures were made from ground jasper or serpentine (both green minerals) in water and from ground carob in fermented honey. An overnight treatment was made from kohl and goose fat, alternatively a paste mixed from equal parts of green eye paint, honey kohl, lapis lazuli, and ochre, applied to the lids.

Not only were cosmetics important in this life, but also in the next one. Chapter 125 of the *Egyptian Book of the Dead* says: "A man says this speech when he is pure, clean, dressed in fresh clothes, shod in white sandals, painted with eye-paint, anointed with the finest oil of myrrh."

The amount and quality of cosmetics and tools such as palettes and brushes among grave goods shows how seriously the they took their cosmetics. Through life and death, the Egyptians pioneered the art of beauty.

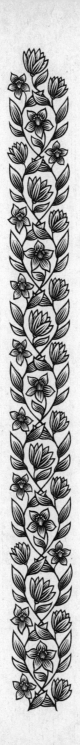

Herb
Crafts

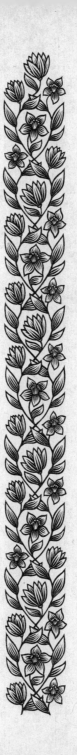

New Hobbies, Recycled Materials

⋙ by Sally Cragin ⋘

Around the time when my son was turning four, he became very interested in color mixing. We read *The Color Kittens* by Margaret Wise Brown (and brilliantly illustrated by Alice and Martin Provenson), and he was captivated with the different shades of secondary colors (green, purple, orange) and what happens when you add additional colors. Somehow, he was happiest finding that all those colors mixed together turned into brown!

When your children are old enough to distinguish colors, why not put a variety of herbs, weeds, and leaves in front of them. Is rosemary light or dark green? Is a sprig of tarragon the same color green as a dandelion weed? Is a buttercup the same yellow as forsythia and daffodil? This requires some discrimination, and you can work on concepts such as light or dark this way.

The great outdoors can provide fun lessons for all seasons, with easy crafts using natural and recycled materials. Although finding useful items is relatively easy, organizing them is a bit more difficult. That's why the overarching principle for me is simplicity. I have been slowly collecting plastic drawers to store our excess inventory, and I try to keep materials of one variety (seashells, seashell fragments for mosaic) in one drawer. (This is the type of activity that a mom with more OCD (obsessive-complusive disorder) than I possess would flourish with!) Also, as a practical matter, I learned with my young son that paints and markers should be kept in the top drawer! We also have lower drawers with broken appliance pieces and jar tops and various bits and pieces to make "machines" and contraptions. We keep ribbons and yarn in one drawer, collage paper in another, and so on. (And we can always use more drawers!)

Spring Crafts

Yes, April showers are definitely for real, and you can make a quickie rainstick as soon as you use that last paper towel. (Here's a hint from the Cheeseparing Family: When you use a paper towel to mop up water or something else that's not noxious, you can let it dry and reuse it. We have a ceramic jar for our still-useful paper towels, which are then usually used for more serious cleaning like stovetop or tidying up after the cat with the secretive hairball habit.)

Homemade Rainstick

You need an empty paper towel or aluminum-foil tube, a couple of feet of aluminum foil, some dried beans, two elastic bands, feathers, ribbons, and other decorative elements. Painting your rainstick ahead of time is a fine idea, but not a requirement.

First, scrunch up the aluminum foil into a long snake about three times as long as the tube. Make it as tight and narrow as you can. Wind the snake around a broomstick so you have a coil as long as your tube. Cap one end of your tube—you can use an old balloon with the end cut off and fasten it with a rubber band, a couple of layers of foil, or stiff paper. Squeeze the foil snake into the tube, so you have a spiral. Pour in one-third to one-half cup of dried beans, popcorn, pebbles, or anything small and rattly. Cap the other end, turn upside down and voilà: "It's raining, it's pouring, the old man is snoring, he bumped his head and went to bed and didn't get up in the morning."

Grassy Hiding Place

Certain containers are forever linked with certain products: The original detergent bottles were designed to look like women's torsos. (Ivory soap still is, actually). Lemon juice usually comes in a dazzling dark-green plastic bottle that gave me a quirky idea for a craft. Take one lemon juice bottle, remove label by soaking, and cut in half crosswise. Cut the remaining cylinder into "grass" with blades no more than one-quarter inch wide. When you have completed this fringe, immerse the plastic in a kettle of boiling water. Get ready to fish this out within a minute or so because the plastic will melt and curl, making a very interesting hiding place for little creatures. We use ours for homemade Easter bunnies made from pipe cleaners and beads, but you could also put a miniature Thanksgiving turkey inside.

Butterfly Crafts

The days get longer and nature blooms in full this season. Planting butterfly-friendly plants such as butterfly bush, elfin herb, porterweed, and golden dewdrop can enhance your garden, and if you're fortunate enough to have milkweed, look for orange monarch butterflies. But even without a garden, an outdoor light can be a gathering place for a wide variety of interesting flying insects. Bear in mind that your child will replicate your response, so if you are a squeamish squealer, you'll probably pass that along to your offspring! Of course, you can make your own instant butterflies by using a round coffee filter (flattened). You can paint with watercolor or poster paint. Buying a bunch of cheap eyedroppers is an excellent investment because you can use them to drop food-coloring solutions onto your filters (always do this craft on an oil cloth or layers of newspaper). Once your filters are dry, you can accordion-fold butterflies and clip with a clothespin painted green or a large paperclip.

Summer Crafts

May Basket

The complete May basket tradition includes filling the basket with sweets and treats and leaving it anonymously on the door-step of one's beloved. All you need for an easy May basket is a white plastic cup and some pipe cleaners. You can have your little one tear bits of colored tissue and glue them on in a mosaic, while older children may be able to cut a "fringe of grass" to glue around the bottom. If you have access to birchbark, wrap a thin layer around the cup. Use one pipe cleaner for a handle and twist real leaves or evergreen needles around the handle with the other pipe cleaner. Use a nail to make two holes in the top opposite one another and voilà! If you select a cup large enough, you can put in seed packets (your own or store-bought).

Bubble Prints

If your child is old enough to "blow" rather than suck through a straw, you can have fun creating colored prints. You'll need some tempera paint, a liquid dish soap, and lots of paper and drinking straws. Put newspaper on the table and lay out some pie pans. In separate cups, you can mix a half cup of water and a generous squirt of soap. Add a tablespoon or so of paint, mix together, and pour into a pie pan. Put the straw into the pie pan, blow until you get a healthy froth and then gently put a piece of paper on your "bubble mountain." Press gingerly and then lift up. You'll have pictures of bubbles. This makes a great wrapping paper for small objects. The trick is preparation so you can have a large work area that includes extra space for the paper to dry.

Firework Pictures

When our son was very small, we discovered that "fireworks" didn't have to use matches. You can make fireworks by wrapping streamers on the end of a stick and hurling into the yard (away from anyone's face, thank you very much). You can also make a fireworks picture by using a pine-needle brush and some black paper. Dip the "brush" into brightly colored paint and sweep across the paper. Or draw stars with colored chalk on dark paper and smear with a fingertip. Another variant is the "starry night" picture, which is best with a child who's old enough to distinguish between a toothbrush you use on your teeth and a toothbrush you use on crafts. Dip a discarded toothbrush into white or silver paint, and "flick" with a thumb across black paper.

Fern Prints

These are quick and easy. Use a sponge brush to paint the underside of a fern and then gently put a piece of paper on top. Smooth with a brayer (small hand-held roller) or the heel of your hand and lift off the paper. If you make enough of these, you can turn them into tree-shaped Christmas cards by adding a star on top.

Dinosaur Fern Park

Every time I turn around it seems there's a tiny little plastic toy underfoot. Many of these are dinosaurs, and one temporary solution for these critters is to construct your own Jurassic Park. Any carton turned on its side will do, or just salvage a flat piece of Styrofoam. Paint it green or brown and poke holes with a bamboo skewer. You can "plant" ferns and other greenery and then have your child place all the little dinos among the wilderness. This is also fun in a sandbox.

Collage Garden

Somewhere along life's journey, we inherited an enormous bag of fabric scraps, many dating from the '70s and '80s. Flower prints were a motif, and most of these remnants were so tiny and made of such ghastly artificial fabrics (remember Dacron?) that you couldn't use them for patchwork. At the time, my son enjoyed drawing lines on paper, so I thought, "why not make a collage garden?" I cut out lots of squares and rectangles of the prints, and we had a jolly time pasting them on paper. Afterward, Christopher drew lines around them for "paths." We've also added paths by streaking a glue-stick on the paper and sprinkling sand.

Autumn Crafts

No vegetable comes close to the mighty pumpkin for holiday hegemony in October, so you can go with the flow by creating pumpkin crafts.

Fun with Seeds

Pumpkin seeds are delicious when roasted (oil pan, clean the seeds, add some salt or salty topping, and roast in a 350-degree F. oven or toaster oven until golden brown), but you can also save and dry them for presents.

Mosaic

Pumpkin seeds are big enough to use for a mosaic. If you still have some watermelon seeds left over you can make a design that uses light/dark. Perhaps a skunk? Or a tree with a shadow? Or use the seeds for a collage. Generally, I think food should be food and crafts should be crafts, but recently I was at a natural-foods grocery store and was enchanted by the range of colors that lentils come in. Perfect mosaic material, with pumpkin seeds for a border.

Seed Packets

The Shakers of New England were the first group to manufacture commercial seed packets on a large scale and you can follow in their footsteps by using summer seeds to make stocking stuffers for friends and family who garden. You can make your own seed packet by taking apart a gift-card envelope and tracing the outline on homemade paper. Fold along lines and decorate before gluing. You can get a little assembly line going for kids who like to draw and glue. Hand lettering is always adorable, or make copies of preprinted designs on a copy machine. A teaspoon of marigold seeds, hollyhock seeds, pumpkin seeds, or squash seeds makes a thoughtful present.

"Hand" Made Turkey

Trace your child's hand on paper, and glue bay leaves on the fingers for feathers. If you use cardboard, you can put a thin layer of white glue on and sprinkle various spices—paprika and cayenne are bright orange, while spices like allspice and cinnamon could be used for contrast. Once the turkey is dry, be sure you put a hole on the tip of the middle finger so you can hang it in the window.

Winter Crafts

Just as the pumpkin obliterates many other images for October, so does the Yule log roll over December's images. Generally, we get moving on the homemade presents around Thanksgiving, and I always like to create in bulk for many family and friends. If you can launch your child toward the idea of making presents, you stand a chance of defusing the rampant materialism that seems inevitable in much of Western culture. But the other crucial step is not overextending yourself. You can spend days making spicy pecans or homemade truffles, but if you don't enjoy it—nor does your child—no one wins. Best to keep this season as simple as you can. We open Christmas cards during the dinner hour after we've eaten so we can enjoy them on the table before paperclipping them to ribbons.

And once the holiday is over, there are always outdoor crafts (see hangers and vases below) and indoor crafts which replicate a snowy landscape. Salt has been a useful craft item for us.

Snow Picture

Put a half cup of salt in a container and add just enough warm water until you have a slurry. Paint "snowscapes" on black construction paper. You can also draw a picture of a house and green trees and then "cover" them with snow. What to do with the leftover "paint?"

Mysterious Snow Crystals

If you use a clear glass or plastic cup, you can see the crystals more clearly. Use your "snow picture" salt solution or just start with a half cup salt added to warm water and stir until dissolved. Tie a washer or bolt onto the end of a string. Wind the string around a chopstick or pencil which you suspend across the top of the clear cup filled with salt solution. As the water evaporates, the crystals grow—they will also grow on the sides of the cup.

Icy Stained-Glass Window Hangers and Vases

This isn't an herbal craft exactly, but you can throw a variety of objects, like pine needle branches and juniper berries into the following projects for interesting results. Or drape red ribbons for a Valentine's tribute.

Window Hangers

First, make sure you have space in your freezer for a pie plate. Grease the pan with oil and then fill he pan halfway with water. Drape a ribbon or decorative twine across the pie plate so that one loop hangs over the edge and the other ends dangle clear of the bottom. Add whatever decorative elements you want, bearing in mind that your creation will melt eventually and you probably don't want sparkly glitter on the grass. Why not try evergreen branches, ribbons, star anise or even strips of colorful cloth? Put in freezer overnight. Hang outside when it's cold enough and enjoy your icy decorations!

Icy Vases

You can make these in clean milk cartons, although a metal or hard plastic container will keep its shape. You'll need lots of interesting long twigs and branches. Fill the container with water, arrange branches (checking to see what fits in the freezer first). Freeze, remove from cold storage, and let thaw just enough to slide out your "vase." Avoid rounded containers or any mold where the top is narrower than the bottom.

Valentine Time

We made a garland last year with a discarded set of playing cards, red heart cutouts, and glued-on rose petals. Remove all the hearts from the deck, punch holes in two corners, thread on red ribbon. Make large red cardstock hearts with various items glued or taped to the front and make a design: perhaps two playing cards, a large heart, two playing cards, a small heart, and so on. Very decorative to hang on the hearth or front door.

Hot Spiced Chocolate Adapted from a Mexican Recipe

March can still have cold days in many parts, and every child is up for a cup of "hot choklit." You may want to go easy on the cloves for the little ones and supervise the stove activity.

Mix together in a paste: two-thirds cup cocoa powder, two-thirds cup sugar, one teaspoon cinnamon, a pinch of clove, and a half cup milk. Heat three cups of milk on the stovetop over medium heat and whisk in your cocoa mixture. This makes a nice froth, so ladle into cups when it's ready. Add a cinnamon stick for ornamentation.

Spice Bag Decorations

You can make these in a square of muslin, but the herbs look very pretty in organza bags. Obviously, the ingredients can vary depending on what's on hand, and making a collection of these is a good way for little ones to practice counting and measuring. Put into one bag:

One to three cinnamon sticks, a tablespoon of cardamom, a tablespoon of cloves, one crushed nutmeg (put into paper bag and reduce to fragments), one or two star anise, mandarin orange peel, and pine sprigs to fill out the bag. You can make a label to attach to a holiday ribbon that explains: "Decorative spice bag. Hang from tree or drop into boiling water for a spicy perfume."

Anytime Avocations

Finally, no craft essay is complete without clay. This versatile substance is ideal for developing fine motor skills to prepare children for writing—and it's fun. We like this recipe a lot and if you add food coloring you can get very pale colors. When this clay is hard, it's rock-hard with a lustrous finish. And it will keep a surprisingly long time in a plastic bag in the fridge. Stir together two cups baking soda and one cup cornstarch. In a saucepan, add one and a half cups water, stirring well. Cornstarch loves to make lumps, so if you're inspired, run it through a sifter first. Cook this mixture over very low heat with occasional stirring for about ten minutes, maybe a little less. Eventually it will look like mashed potatoes. Remove the pan from the heat and when the clay is cool enough to handle, turn out on a floured board. You can knead this clay and add more cornstarch as needed. You don't want this too wet or it gets very floppy. Creations can be air-dried overnight or longer.

Herbal Home Care

※ by Janice Sharkey ※

Herbs have played an all-encompassing role in the household since medieval times. Very few herbs were cultivated purely for their beauty alone. In an age without off-the-shelf household sprays and cleaners, ancient folk had to venture into their garden to find a way of keeping their living space clean and pleasant. Almost every flower and herb had some use, if only to make a scented carpet to discourage insects and help mask the strong odors that were a part of everyday medieval life before modern-day plumbing and waste disposal. Early medical books often lumped the care of the body with the care of the home because both contributed to an overall sense of well-being.

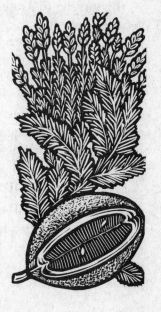

Everything that nature provided was used. The produce from the herbal garden contributed toward making cleansers, bleaches, and conditioners; cut flowers were used for bedrooms, pillows, and sweet-linen bags. Our ancient ancestors would use such things as smudge sticks or pomanders to freshen the air. Used sparingly, they brought the fresh aroma of the forest and herb garden into the home.

Let us take the modern shop's cleaning products out of their packets and back into nature's world from where they can be harvested in their optimum state, free of added preservatives and other man-made chemicals. Take for example lemon, which is sharp in taste, yet cooling and acidic. Its skin contains an insect-repellent and a strong oily antiseptic. There are many ways we can use these qualities: the mild acids can clean metal, bleach linen, whiten skin, and lighten hair; the peel can disinfect, repel insects, discourage moths, or be used as an antiseptic; the seeds can kill parasitic worms and also produce another lemon tree. And if that wasn't enough, it is full of vitamin C to keep our immune system fighting fit.

By turning to Mother Nature's herbal cleaners, we can use gentle cleansers and vastly reduce the harmful chemicals that lurk in many mass-produced household cleaners. Not only do we benefit by breathing in good natural air, reducing the risk of asthma and curbing the intake of yet more chemicals into the body, so too, we do not "dump" and dispose of harmful chemicals into the water and the ecosystem. Herbal cleaners are nature's way of striking a balance to live practically, cleanly, and give our senses a spring clean.

Household Cleaners

Our kitchens often harbor a multitude of bacteria, which, if left to fester, could do us harm. Natural herbal cleaners don't just mask bad smells in a kitchen, their properties actually fight to cleanse the air and surfaces they touch. When used correctly, they are harmless and safe to touch and use on cooking surfaces. Besides food-preparation surfaces harboring germs, the steam from cooking also emits tiny molecules of fat into the air. What you'll need is an herbal cleaner that cuts through grease and deodorizes, leaving the kitchen as fresh and appetizing as the dinner you have slaved over. Try some of these kitchen germ busters:

Bacteria Busters

These can be used in the bathroom and kitchen and include clove, lemon, pine, eucalyptus, lavender, thyme, lime, and grapefruit. You may have noticed most are citrus fruits due to their antifungal and antiviral properties as well as their fresh fragrance. Eucalyptus is one herb with disinfectant qualities that actually improves with age, so its shelf life is unlimited. Some of these herbs cannot be grown easily, but their fruits can be bought and the oils extracted quite cheaply.

Windows

Smear marks can often be left on windows, but can also be easily remedied. Add a drop of lime or lemon juice to a crumpled sheet of paper and polish the windows. This gets any streaky marks off and adds a sparkling finish.

Bed Linen and Washing

Add a drop of lavender or lemongrass essential oil to your linen during the wash or while being dried or even when stored. If winter colds and flu have struck the household, put a drop of eucalyptus, pine, or rosemary into the wash water. These oils are especially beneficial on bed linen to counter viruses and bacteria; they also help relieve coughs and catarrh. If suffering from insomnia, marjoram, chamomile, or orange blossom will help you sleep if used when rinsing nightwear and bedding. Why not infuse clothes tumbling in the dryer? Just add two drops of an herbal oil onto a spare piece of material and pop in with the clothes. For freshness, try lavender or rosemary. To add a little romantic aroma to the bed sheets, put two drops of jasmine or rose oil onto the bed sheets and let the scent circulate the bedroom.

Rugs

Years ago, people put aromatic grasses under their rugs and mats so the scent would be released to freshen the room. Many people have their rooms fully carpeted, so a more practical idea is to make your own homemade carpet freshener, which can include ingredients such as talc, kaolin, essential oils, and bicarbonate of soda. Allow one tablespoonful of each and add to a blender before including one drop of your chosen fragrance, such as lavender.

Vacuum Cleaner

To keep a vacuum smelling fresh, place six to eight drops of lemon, orange, lavender, or pine essential oil on a cotton-wool ball and put it in your vacuum cleaner bag, which will also help eradicate dustiness. If you are using disposable bags, simply put a drop of the favorite herbal oil directly onto the bag.

Kitchen Germ Busters

Where food is prepared can harbor a multitude of germs. To banish these, put one drop of herbal oil, ideally lemon, directly onto a cloth or stir seven drops of lavender, lime, grapefruit, pine, or thyme into the rinse water.

Washing Floors

Try a synergistic blend of homemade, antibacterial disinfectant that leaves a delightful fragrance with the added benefit of being mood enhancing. Let's face it—we need a boost to see us through the monotonous job of housework. Try this recipe: put 8 drops of herbal oil into 600 milliliters of water and get mopping. Why not use the same blend and convert it into a spray that can be used in all sorts of surfaces around the house? If storing this herbal mixture, put in a clean, brown glass bottle and store away from light and heat.

Tea-Towel

As many washes don't reach boiling point, they fail to kill off the microbes that stay on tea-towels. So soak them in a bowl of boiling water and add one drop of eucalyptus, thyme, tea tree or, my favorite, lavender. Leave to soak for a while before putting into the usual machine wash.

Add Herbs to Dishwashers

Before switching on the cycle, add two drops of lemon juice into the container—smell the difference and be assured that every dish will be naturally clean.

Furniture Polish

Beeswax polish is the ideal furniture polish because it's natural and nourishing to wood. You can make your own by buying plain beeswax from beekeepers or good hardware stores. Just add the herbal oil of your choice and thoroughly mix into the beeswax before polishing.

Making Your Own Soaps

Even though it might seem like a messy chore at first, making your own soaps has many benefits and leads to a lot of satisfaction—and who knows, maybe an idea for giving personalized fragrant gifts to friends and family. However, one thing is certain: you will know what goes into your soap and can therefore be proactive in reducing the chance of contracting skin allergies due to contact with chemical fragrances found in some soaps. You can even shape your soap in a special mold that gives it that quirky individual quality. The world's your oyster when it comes to choice of fragrance for your soap—you don't even have to stick to just one herbal oil.

How about a mixture of tangy grapefruit, lime, and lemon (one drop each) that helps cleanse and clear toxins not only from the body, but your mind as well? For a more relaxing and calming blend, try six drops of lavender and two drops of geranium, which is soothing and good for replenishing the skin. To use as a base for your soap, acquire a cake of pure soap and add oatmeal and olive, sweet almond, or jojoba oil. Bring to a boil water that is half the volume of the grated soap. Put this in a double-boiler or a bowl over a pot of boiling water and allow the grated soap to melt slowly. Give it a stir until it is quite sticky and then remove from the heat. Leave until it is starting to set, at which point you add your chosen herbal oils. Now mix well. After this, scoop out the soap and put into a suitable mold or shape it by hand if you prefer. You can be creative and use old soapboxes or small containers but make sure they are oiled or lined with greaseproof paper. Leave until well set and then turn out the soap. Dress up the soaps with ribbon and colored tissue paper if giving them as gifts.

Perfumed Pillows

Why not take a leaf out of the medieval housewife's book? Allow your head to once again lay back on a perfumed pillow smelling of sweet aromas and herbal sachets full of a potpourri of essences that will help heal and cleanse your body and mind. Day pillows would release a portion of their fragrance each time someone leaned back on them, and sachets were slipped into drawers, cupboards, shoes, and boots to keep them all sweet smelling. So first, get a piece of material stitched along three sides and add fresh-dried herbs or spices. For enhancing sleep, use lavender, chamomile, valerian, or nutmeg. Cushions can have their fragrance matched to the scent of the room such as geranium. When you have made your choice of herbs, stitch up the fourth side of the sachet, insert into the pillow or cushion, and let the aroma begin its magic.

Smudge Sticks

A smudge stick is a collection of herbs tied up and used to freshen the air, clear unpleasant smells, and ward off insects. Used sparingly, they bring a touch of the forest and garden into the home.

Just pick sprigs of fresh, healthy young herb leaves such as sage, thyme, rosemary, fennel and their stalks, or choose something from the forest such as pine or cypress. Hold the sprigs tightly and tie with thread or string. Leave the sticks to dry naturally over a few weeks in a dry place. To use, hold the end about five centimeters above a candle flame. It will take time, but the end will become red and smolder, releasing a thin trail of fragrant smoke. Some oily herbs may splutter and spit oil as they burn. When the smudge stick has done its work, put it out carefully and trim the end so it is ready for immediate use the next time you need it.

Pomanders

These balls of fragrance hold their aroma for years with lemon and oranges being the most popular base to begin making one. Spear either with cloves or aromatic seed such as fennel, cumin, and caraway. Make small, shallow holes in the peel, not deep enough to pierce the flesh. Put cloves in the holes, in rows and patches or at random. To finish the pomander, just rub it with ground cloves and salt to preserve it. Then hang up and allow it to dry naturally.

Grow Your Own Stock Herbs

Most herbs love sunshine, so find a sunny spot for lavender, rosemary, and thyme. Even if you don't have a garden, plant them in pots at doorways and patios—any place where the sun will release their wonderful "brush me" fragrance. If you have space, eucalyptus is a great herb to plant; although fast growing, it's evergreen all year round and its "crush me" leaves are very versatile for use around the home. Scented geraniums are great houseplants helping to naturally release lovely aromas to lighten the spirit of a room. Hardy geraniums are tough plants against pests and also good for harvesting into herbal remedies.

Drawing on the Past

Why not learn from our ancient ancestors? Walk into a medieval kitchen and you would find on display a rich harvest of herbal diversity—leaves, stems, bark, roots, tubers, seeds, and also fruit. These would be put to good use in naturally cleansing our homes and transforming where we live into a fragrant bouquet. (These organic cleansers and aromas cannot be replicated by anything we could purchase off the store shelf.) So let your herbal garden be your store to banish harmful bacteria from your home.

Plant-Based Fabric Dyes

~ by Calantirniel ~

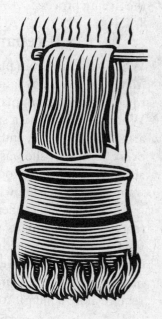

Plants have been a main source of textile dyes for hundreds of years—that is, until the Industrial Age, when chemical dyes were invented to create more colorfastness and color accuracy while producing a much wider range of colors than ever before possible. The process also became easier and less costly, all but pushing plant-based dying into antiquity.

Why revive this practice now? There are many people who wish to live in harmony with the cycles of Earth—they eat vegan, organic foods, use solar power and other alternative energies for their houses and cars, and wear natural fabrics—where chemical dyes do not have a place. This article is intended as a starting point, as the process is not difficult. If you are open-minded regarding your results, you just might have some fun, and be proud to wear an item that you have imparted with a plant's vibrational energy!

The colors most difficult (or expensive) to achieve are on the cooler end of the spectrum: blues, purples, and brighter reds. Plants like indigo and woad cannot be covered here, since their process is entirely different and involves fermentation. However, with simple plant material from your yard, hiking trip, kitchen, grocery, or herb store, you can create wonderful shades in the warmer end of the spectrum: yellows and golds, oranges, rusts, tans, browns, and olive-type greens—even black! You can also achieve a certain level of success with the cooler spectrum colors.

Fabric Selection

Generally, it is easier to dye animal-sourced fabrics, like silk and washed wool, rather than plant-based fabrics. However, I have had wonderful results with cotton and hemp. Note that the chosen fabric needs to be in a clean, natural state and receptive to the dyeing process.

Preparing the Dye Bath

When gathering your plant materials (see the "Colors and Plant Materials" list below), make sure you are not externally allergic to your chosen plant matter by boiling a small amount in water. When cool, apply to a small patch of skin on the inside of your arm, allow it to dry, and observe for reactions over the next day or so. Some may show as early as a few minutes—wash with non-allergenic soap and choose a different plant. For example, black walnut hulls are a known allergen.

After making smaller pieces of your collected plant material (chopping or tearing is usually enough; the plant pieces should float around freely in the dye bath water), place it into a large ceramic or stainless steel pot with water, bring to a boil, and if needed, turn off heat and let sit overnight (some plant materials require more boiling). You are done boiling or soaking when plant material looks exhausted of color and the color is instead imparted in the water. Remove plant material with a strainer or cheesecloth, then discard. If you use a copper or an aluminum pot, be prepared for color change because water boiled in these will accumulate the residual metals of the pot (and could even dye the pot!). If you are unsure of how much plant material to use, err on the side of too much color because the item will fade with every wash. I usually find a good proportion by filling the pot halfway with plant matter, then add water up until the pot is three-fourths full. You can also add more water and not feel too bad about diluting it too much. Lighter shades in the same color family can be diluted even more—for instance, plant material for creating magenta can be diluted further to make a light pink color.

Beginners should stick to one type of plant material at first. (For example, use a pot of carrot tops only rather than a combination of green materials). After gaining some experience, you can blend plant materials for the same color, and even plant materials of different colors to create a blended color. Test a small fabric swatch of each individual plant material first so you have an idea of what to expect when blending together. Even then, you may still be surprised, which is part of the beauty and splendor of nature's chemistry!

Upon gathering your plant material, you will most likely need to add a "mordant" to the dye bath to create colorfastness. Alum (aluminum ammonium sulfate) is the best and most readily available, or you can use a blend of three parts alum to one part cream of tartar to brighten and soften fabric. White vinegar has also been used, but can dull the color. Some plant materials, like turmeric, meadowsweet roots, and black walnut hulls do not need a mordant to create colorfastness due to constituents present within the plant that adhere the plant's inherent color onto the fabric. However, should you choose to use a mordant, know that it may change the resultant color. If you wish to create a color in the ashier part of the cooler range (for example, to turn a light brown to a bluish gray), you can try iron as a mordant rather than alum, but it is not as readily available (although an old technique is to throw some rusting nails into the dye bath or use a rusty cast iron pot that you don't mind getting stained). The proportion needed is one teaspoon mordant per quart of plant dye solution. If you decide to use vinegar as mordant, use one-quarter cup per quart. Dissolve thoroughly.

A Walk Through the Process

If you wish to make a light-golden brown color, collect onion skins from yellow and/or brown onions. Fill the dye bath pot halfway with crushed onion skins. Then add water until the dye pot is three-quarters full.

Boil and/or soak until the color is in the water and absent from the onion skins. When this happens, strain out and discard the onion skins, and keep the colored water in the pot. You can add more water if it is needed.

Now, add the mordant to the dye bath. In this case, it is one teaspoon of alum or the blend mentioned above per quart of dye path. Dissolve thoroughly.

Dyeing the Fabric

Thoroughly wet the clean, oil-free item to be dyed with barely hot water before placing into the dye bath. Make sure the entire item is immersed and that the dye can easily reach every part of the item so that coloring is consistent, not splotchy. Allow to simmer on the stove for an hour, stirring periodically; or if you prefer (especially in a case where heat would destroy the plant dye, particularly the yellows and reds), you can let it sit covered all day in the hot sun, stirring periodically. (Be careful with wool, which might shrink with rapid temperature change.) Rinse the item in water—hotter water at first, then cooler water until it rinses nearly clear. Some prefer to further "set" color in water with white vinegar (use one-fourth cup to a quart of water), but beware that this can dull some colors, so test it out first. Then you can wash in cool water and mild soap (with a few drops of a pleasant essential oil, like lavender, if dyeing materials had an unpleasant odor); rinse in cool water, and you are done! Notice any color changes while the item is drying. You may be pleasantly surprised at your results, but if you are not overjoyed, keep trying different mixes until they work—again, all part of the fun! Make sure you keep thorough notes for referencing later. For maintenance of the item, color will stay longer if you wash in a gentle cleanser in cooler water. If you wish to lighten the item without washing, try laying it in the sun on dry green grass, turning over as needed, until the desired color is evident.

Colors and Plant Materials

This is only intended as a starting place (tumeric, onion skins, henna, beets, and coffee are the easiest materials for beginners to work with), as you can use a wide variety of plants, depending on what is available for you—and part of the fun is seeing what colors in fact do arise from different plant materials. Try many types of leaves, flowers, fruits/berries, hulls, barks, roots, seeds, and even lichens. Break them down first by chopping or tearing into small enough pieces to fit loosely in the dye bath. When you get more comfortable, you may even wish to mix different plant matter to achieve even more colors through a process involving overdyeing a number of times to achieve a particular color. (When overdyeing, start with the dark color, let the fabric dry, then re-dye to achieve the desired tone.) This entire process gives one a great respect for the textile dyers of commerce in the past. The beauty of color, colorfastness, and color consistency were all factors in keeping them in business. This is not just science—it is an art! Have fun creating!

Greens: Azalea leaves, carrot tops, poplar leaves, spinach leaves, lamb's quarters (goosefoot), tansy leaves, and black-eyed Susan flowers. Or a two-step process, dyeing with blue first, then overdyeing with yellow. Some yellow plant materials may work with iron mordant.

Yellows and Golds: Turmeric (no mordant needed), annato seeds, fustic, saffron (expensive), dock leaves and roots, goldenrods, dandelions, marigolds, zinnias and other yellow flowers, ragweed leaves, mullein, wild mustard, parsley, alder and birch leaves, sunflower (flowers and whole seeds), onion skins (yellow to brown), and a variety of leaves, particularly in autumn.

Oranges and Rusts: Carrots or beta-carotene powder, henna (use lemon or other citrus juice, wine, or vinegar as mordant), and plant materials from "yellows and golds" mixed with plant materials for "reds, magentas, pinks and purples." Or use a two-step process; dyeing with red first, then overdyeing with yellow.

Reds, Magentas, Pinks, and Purples: Madder root, Brazilwood, paprika, pomegranate berries, caesalpinia bark, black currant berries, blackberries, mulberries, wild grapes, alkanet, red cabbage, logwood, hibiscus flowers, dandelion roots, and beets (use juice or powder).

Tans and Browns: Acorns (whole), cherry bark and branches, pine cones, birch leaves, hawthorn berries, hickory hulls and branches, walnut bark and hulls, onion skins (brown to dark red), coffee, tea, and the darker leaves of autumn.

Black: Logwood, oak galls, black walnut hulls (no mordant needed), meadowsweet roots (no mordant needed), blackberry leaves, or any plant materials in "browns" using iron mordant.

Grays: Bayberry leaves, blackberry shoots, sumac berries, or any plant material for "tan" using iron mordant.

Blues: Elderberries, spiderwort flowers, red cabbage, tomato leaves and stems, or the purplish plant materials in "reds, magentas, pinks, and purples" using iron mordant. (Indigo and woad use a vastly different dying procedure that includes fermentation.)

Herb-Filled Poppets

❧ by Suzanne Ress ❧

Poppet is the old-fashioned English word for "doll." It comes from the French *poupée*, and is closely related to the word *puppet*—a human-manipulated figure.

Historically, all over the world (and until relatively recently in Western civilization) dolls, or poppets, have always been handmade. They could be made from almost anything, including clay, wax, animal bone, straw, corn-husk, scraps of woven fabric, and wood, depending on available materials.

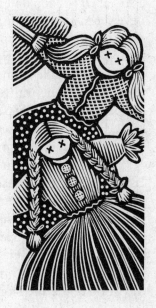

Most people think of modern man-ufactured dolls as toys for children, but in the past, poppets were often made for purposes of image, or sympathetic, magic. Especially common in many cultures were fertility poppets, but there were also poppets for healing, success, love, and protection.

The first known magical doll figures were the mother goddesses that date back to at least 23,000 BC. Found in archeological dig sites, these were small female figures carved out of rock, with relatively huge breasts and bellies, and were, most probably, used as earth fertility charms. One of the most well known is the "Venus of Willendorf," a limestone carving that stands 4¾ inches tall, and was unearthed in the early 1900s in Austria.

Babylonians made figures of their enemies and then destroyed them as a form of protective magic. The idea of protecting yourself against someone you feared by piercing his image (the poppet) with pins, needles, or nails, goes back at least as far as ancient Egypt and Mesopotamia, about 3000 to 4000 years BC.

Although sticking pins and nails into an image of one's enemy doesn't sound very kind, it is one form of sympathetic magic—the image takes on part of the identity, or sympathizes with, the one it represents. This sort of magic has been practiced using both human and animal images for protection, love, and healing for a very long time, but the distorted concept of sticking pins into a so-called voodoo doll to harm or even kill another person has never been a socioculturally acceptable practice anywhere.

Ancient Greek poppets were called *kolossoi* and were used to keep ghosts or evil spirits away, or to bind two lovers together. These were made of metal, wood, or clay, and, in the case of protection magic, thirteen pins or nails were driven into the poppet to figuratively paralyze the feared one's faculties such as sight, hearing, feeling, etc. If known, the name of the evil spirit or ghost was inscribed on the left side of the figure.

In pre-Christian times, Druids made corn dollies from the last sheaf of wheat to ensure a successful harvest for the following year. During the sixteenth century in the African Congo basin (a region known for forests), poppets called *Nkondi* were made of wood, with a carved open space in the belly or head for "medicines" composed of fruit, mushrooms, and charcoal. Nkondi were used for divination, as protective figures, or as a means to see into the world of the ancestors.

The infamous voodoo dolls of New Orleans are actually hoodoo dolls from West African slaves' magical practices, and they were used in sympathetic ways similar to those of other ancient religious/magical practices from all over the world. Most likely, white slave owners catching glimpses of these unfamiliar ritual poppets misunderstood their true purpose and the myth was perpetuated from that time.

In modern Wiccan love magic practices, two poppets, each representing one of the potential lovers, are bound together face to face, using red thread or ribbon to symbolize eternal love (as do modern wedding bands).

Besides their historical use as images for sympathetic magic, herb-filled poppets can be used by anyone to scent a drawer, purse, or automobile; keep moths out of closets and chests; as worry pieces to hold onto inside a pocket; or as tiny scented gifts.

When making an herb-filled poppet, you can select the fabric and herbal scents to match the person or décor, make the fabric match the scent (as in green calico for a mint filled poppet), or simply to express a mood.

Herb-filled poppets can be any size, but I have found 3-inches tall to be most practical. Though traditionally most poppets are human shaped, there have always been a few animal-shaped ones, too, so I have included instructions to make a basic animal poppet as well.

A Small Herb-Filled Poppet

This poppet is only 3 inches tall, and its body form can be customized to represent a male or female, even a specific person, if you wish. The end result is an aromatic, portable talisman that can be carried in a glove compartment, purse, or in a pocket as a "worry piece," releasing its herbal scents as it is secretly rubbed and handled.

You will need tightly woven medium-weight cotton fabric—the kind often used for quilters' squares is fine, though flannel works well, too. If you want to make a realistic-looking poppet, choose a solid color fabric in the skin tone of your choice. Otherwise, you can make a flowered, checkered, plaid, or calico print poppet. For each poppet the basic supplies you will need are a 4 × 8-inch rectangle of fabric, threads in various colors, scissors, a needle, dried herbs, and several cotton balls.

On a piece of paper, measure a 4-inch square and draw a simple human stick figure in it. Then draw an outline about ¼ inch around the outside of all the stick figure lines except the legs, where you will only draw around the outsides of the stick figure legs, so it seems as if your figure is wearing a long skirt. The ends of the figure's arms should touch the sides of the rectangle, his head the top, and the hem of his "skirt" the bottom.

Cut out your paper pattern. Fold your 4 × 8-inch fabric rectangle in half to make a 4-inch square, and pin the pattern to the fabric. Cut along the outside of the pattern, and unpin.

If you wish to embroider features such as eyes, nose, mouth, belly button, etc., on your poppet, do it now before sewing him up. Keep in mind that you will lose (to seams) a margin of fabric space all around, so do not sew facial features too close to the edges of the fabric.

Embroidering the Details

Before embroidering the face, draw the features onto the fabric with a pencil. A single strand of thread in a color one or two shades darker than your fabric makes a good nose, belly button, and un-madeup eyelids. Use small French knots and simple line stitches. Slightly darker shades work well for eyebrows and made-up eyelids. Use pinks or reds for lips, and blacks, blues, greens, browns, or ambers for eyes. Try embroidering open lips and sewing on a tiny white or gold seed bead or two to represent teeth. Don't forget to embroider beards and mustaches, if desired. A small heart shape can be sewn in purple, red, pink, or gold thread in the center of the poppet's chest. Embroider any other markings such as tattoos or random or meaningful symbols on the body, or leave it plain.

If you are not skilled at embroidery, you can draw the face on with permanent fine-tipped markers, or leave it featureless.

Once you are satisfied with the details (or lack of them), use tiny hand stitches to sew, decorated sides inward, close to the outer edges of the fabric. Leave the entire bottom edge of the poppet unsewn. Sew the seams under the arms and on both sides of the neck a second time to reinforce them.

Using the eraser end of a small pencil, and a pair of tweezers if necessary, carefully turn your poppet right-side out.

Now you are ready to stuff him.

Stuffing the Poppet

First, stuff the head and neck with surgical cotton or cotton balls. Tear off small pieces of cotton and slowly push them into the head using the blunt end of a pencil. Pack the cotton tightly, and when the head and neck look well filled out, stuff the poppet's arms the same way.

You will need between ⅓ and ½ cup of dried herb blend to finish stuffing your small poppet. Use your fingers to push in as much as will fit, then turn the raw edges of fabric at the opening narrowly to the inside and sew the poppet closed.

To finish the poppet a small wig can be made, using any variety of yarn, embroidery floss, metallic craft "angel hair," steel wool, synthetic doll hair, ostrich plume, real human hair left from a haircut, or anything else that strikes your fancy.

For a yarn or floss wig, closely wind it 10 to 20 times around a piece of cardboard whose width is twice the length you wish the poppet's hair to be; for shoulder-length hair, use a 1½- to 2-inch-wide strip of cardboard; for ankle length hair, a 6-inch wide strip. When you've finished winding the yarn, use beige thread to sew through all the yarn or floss at one edge of the cardboard, then sew them twice more, to make a part. Cut the yarn or floss at the opposite edge of the cardboard. Arrange the wig on the poppet's head and sew in place. You can then trim or style the poppet's hair.

One or many necklaces, bracelets, earrings, or anklets can be sewn onto the poppet's neck, wrists, etc. A slender ribbon can be tied around a female poppet's waist to represent a dress, or you can make a tiny cloak by hemming a 5 x 4-inch rectangle of contrasting fabric, gathering one 5-inch edge and sewing it to the poppet at the neck. Other clothes for small poppets are not recommended because too many layers of fabric get in the way of the herbal scent.

A Small Animal-Shaped Poppet

This is a generic animal that can be modified with minor details to represent a dog, cat, donkey, or small horse.

Start with a 4-inch square of paper and draw a line down the center, one line horizontally across about ½ inch from the bottom edge, another horizontal line about 1½ inches from the top edge, and a round head on top. On one side of the head, draw an oval shape representing a muzzle. Now draw a line about a ½ inch out, around the entire stick figure. Cut the pattern out and pin it to a 4 x 8-inch rectangle of fabric folded in half. For an animal poppet you can use any print or appropriately colored medium-weight cotton fabric or fake fur, although this latter is difficult to work with.

Embroider an eye in the center of the round part of each head piece, making sure to embroider the opposite sides of each piece so that when you sew them together, the eyes will both be on the outside of the fabric.

Now sew around all the seams in small stitches close to the edges of the fabric, leaving the animal's "back" open.

Turn the animal right-side out with the help of a small, blunt pencil or similar tool. Stuff the head and legs tightly with small pieces of surgical or cosmetic cotton.

Fill the rest of the animal poppet with a dried herb blend and sew up the back seam, turning the raw edges of the fabric to the inside.

Depending on what animal you wish the poppet to represent, you can make ears from matching or color-coordinated felt scraps, a tail from yarn, embroidery floss, felt, etc. and, if called for, a matching mane. Add embroidered nostrils or whiskers and a slender ribbon around the neck or tail, if desired.

Use your imagination and have fun making your poppets as wild or as sweet as you please.

Drying Herbs and Preparing Aromatic Blends

For the most potent fragrance, herb leaves should be picked or cut just before the plant flowers—this is when the herb will be at the peak of its aromatic or balsamic phase. When gathering flowers you wish to dry, such as chamomile or lavender, the right moment to pick is just as the flowers begin to open. Naturally, not all the herbs and flowers in your garden will be ready for gathering at the same time. In general, most herbs will be ready for harvesting sometime during the months of June, July, or August, but, depending on the age of the individual plant, your climate, and how the season goes, some herbs are ready as early as April and others not until late September.

When they are ready, both leaves and flowers should be gathered, preferably on a clear dry day in the morning after the dew has dried, but before the sun gets too hot. Pinch off tender herbs and flowers such as sage, rose geranium, costmary, bay, basil and Melissa, but use a pocket knife, garden scissors, or boleen (a small scythe used exclusively for herb cutting) to cut tougher stemmed herbs such as hyssop, lavender, mint, hops, chamomile, lemon verbena, rosemary, southernwood, and wormwood, without damaging the plant.

Herbs can be hung in small bunches upside down in an airy room, or laid out on a drying rack, easily made from a wood pallet and a piece of screen (a window screen will work fine). They can also be placed in large woven natural baskets, and small amounts can simply be laid out on a clean dish towel some place where they will not be disturbed. Whichever method you choose, make sure they are not in direct sunlight, since this will cause them to fade and remove much of their aroma. Unless the herbs are hung to dry they should be turned over once every couple of days. Depending on the herb and the weather, it can take anywhere from two days to two weeks to dry thoroughly. When they are ready, the leaves and flower petals will crumble easily between your fingers. Once they are dry, herbs and flowers should be stored whole, loosely packed in glass jars, in a cool dark place such as a pantry or basement.

As soon as you have a good selection of dried herbs and flowers to choose from, you can start experimenting with different aromatic blends for use in specific poppets.

Here are some of my favorite recipes, all of which have self-explanatory uses. To make them, simply combine all dry ingredients, add the essential oil, and mix well.

Lucky Blend: Equal parts peppermint, calamint, and basil plus 2 drops ginger oil. (This blend smells fresh, minty, and a bit like new money.)

Pick-Me-Up: 2 parts rose geranium leaf; 1 part rosemary.

Sweet Dreams: (A soothing and calming scent): 1 part chamomile flowers, ½ part calendula flower petals, and 1 part lemon balm (Melissa).

Awareness Blend: Equal parts thyme, sage, and lavendar.

Wake-Me-Up: Equal parts lemon verbena, marjoram, and spearmint.

Moth Away: Equal parts southernwood and wormwood.

Relax Blend: 1 part hops flowers, 1 part chamomile flowers, ½ part feverfew flowers, and 1 drop valerian oil.

Safe and Away! Blend: Equal parts fennel seed, angelica leaf, and basil leaf.

No More Tears Blend: 1 part bee balm (bergamot), ½ part lemon verbena, ½ part lemon grass, and 1 drop bitter orange oil.

The Four Seasons of Garden Crafts

by Lisa McSherry

As gardeners, we tend to view the long term with more equanimity than most people. No matter if our gardens spread across acres or are limited to scattered containers, we understand that each seed takes its own time to sprout and grow and that there are four definite seasons to the garden's life. Similarly, there are four distinct seasons for crafting things based on what the garden is producing (or has recently produced).

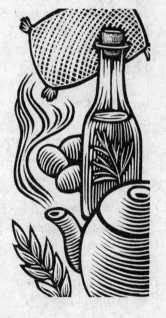

Winter

Winter is a time of warding off the stress of the holiday season and then staying healthy while we wait for the sun to return. This is when we want to take our tonics, make crafts for friends and loved ones, and drink warming teas while we rest and recover.

Healing Teas

As a child I had terrible chest colds lasting for weeks, until my mother created this tea to drink. For years I mixed a jar of these herbs at the beginning of winter and kept the mixture ready to brew at the earliest sign of a cold. Fair warning: Nothing makes this tea taste good, but a little goes a long way, and it works incredibly well.

Chest Cold Tea

1   part mint (peppermint or spearmint)

1   part chamomile

1   part horehound

½   part red clover

½   part coltsfoot

Mix the ingredients well. Place about 1 ounce of the dry herbs into a teapot. Boil water until just bubbling and pour 2 cups over herbs. Cover and let steep, about 15 minutes. Strain and drink. Dosage: ½ cup of tea every 4 hours. You can add honey to ease the taste, but I usually just held my nose, tossed the tea down my throat, and ate a carrot as quickly as I could before I let go of my nose.

Horehound is the major player in this tea as it is an expectorant and soothing for the mucous membranes. The mint and chamomile are present mostly to ease the taste (and they assist the healing properties by calming the muscles and gently opening the nasal passages). Red clover relaxes muscles and eases coughing.

Relaxing Tea

Many wise people have pointed out that the high levels of stress that most of us deal with on a daily basis are a major cause of our ill health. To that end, our most potent weapon against ill health—especially in the dark winter months when it's hard to get the energy flowing—might be taking the time each day for a relaxing cup of tea.

1   part chamomile

½   part raspberry leaf or lemon balm

½   part catnip

½   part passion flower

Mix herbs and store in an airtight jar until ready to use. To brew, heat water just to a boil. Place 2 teaspoons of the herb mixture in a mug and pour in 1 cup of boiling water. Steep 5 minutes, strain, and enjoy.

Chamomile is a mild sedative, as is lemon balm, which is also used as an antidepressant. Catnip is good for the digestive system and passionflower is another plant with sedative properties.

'Forting Up' Against Illness Tea

I know that I often miss out on the first wave of colds that make their way through my office, but somehow the second round always gets me. This tea, taken every day, now helps me avoid even that round.

1   slice fresh ginger, about the thickness of a quarter

1   ¼-inch piece licorice root

1   ¼-inch piece cinnamon stick

1   teaspoon dried parsley

1   clove

1   teaspoon dried orange rind

Bring water just to a boil, pour 1 cup over ingredients. Steep for 5 to 15 minutes, depending on how strong you like it. Strain and enjoy.

Ginger enhances the immune system and licorice has anti-bacterial properties. Cinnamon, of course, is a warming spice and recent research indicates that it helps diabetics in balancing their blood sugar. Parsley is a digestive aid and the orange rind and clove add exotic flavor.

Spring

For most of us, spring can't come soon enough. We want to get into our garden, start planting, and celebrate the warming days.

There are many gardens we can create according to a theme. Most of my gardening has been based on what I can plant in containers (the joys of being a city-living apartment dweller!) and I think this makes theme plantings a lot easier. If a plant isn't getting enough sun or doesn't like its neighbors, it is easy to move the pot to a new location. Here are some thematic gardens I've planted over the years:

Butterfly Bliss

Butterflies are attracted to nectar-producing plants that bloom throughout the season, particularly from mid- to late summer. This means planting flowers that bloom in successive waves.

Perennials: Aster, bee-balm, black-eyed Susan, daylilies, hibiscus, lobelia, phlox, and sage.

Annuals: Cosmos, impatiens, marigold, nasturtium, verbena, and zinnia.

Purple and White

I will confess, this is the garden I planted for Spring 2007. I went for color rather than practicality. Wandering through the nursery it occurred to me that purple and white would make a really nice combination. I planted the flowers in groups along with red-bladed, spiky *Cordyline indivisa* (*Dracaena*) and long trailers of an ivylike plant called moonlit dwarf periwinkle, which has a variegated leaf and produces deep purple flowers.

Purple flowers: Foxglove, delphinium, lobelia, pansy, stock, and sweet pea.

White flowers: Alyssum, honeysuckle, pansy, rose, and sweet pea.

General Purpose

This is a garden for cooking and making healing teas. Plant garlic (not too close to windows or doors—it is a very pungent), peppermint (this plant does very well in a container—it will absolutely take over a garden if planted in the ground), rosemary, lavender, carnation (different varieties have scents ranging from lemon to spice), sage, and basil.

Egg Crafts

It's been a long time since I colored eggs to celebrate the visit by the chocolate-carrying bunny. But since I discovered that it's not necessary to use commercial food dyes, I like to color up a bunch of eggs and decorate them to give away.

The quick way to color eggs is to wrap them in onion skins with twine and hard boil them. When the eggs are cooked, unwrap the twine and carefully remove the skins (they'll be kind of gooey). A random mottling of orangey-brown or purplish tracings will be all over the eggs. To get an even tone, place the onion skins into the water before boiling the eggs.

A longer process involves cooking up dyes and soaking hard-boiled eggs in them. The recipe is basically the same: 1 quart water, 2 tablespoons white vinegar, and the desired dye.

Color	Ingredient	Amount
Blue	Red cabbage leaves	½ head (4 cups, chopped)
Pink	Beets	4 cups, chopped (3 whole)
Yellow	Turmeric	3 tablespoons
Green	Spinach	4 cups, chopped

To make: Place all ingredients for the chosen color into a heavy saucepan and bring to a boil. Reduce heat and simmer 30 minutes. Strain and place dye into a bowl deep enough to cover eggs. Let eggs soak in the dye until they reach the desired color. Color will start to adhere in as little as 5 minutes, but you can let the eggs soak overnight to achieve a deep, dramatic color.

Summer

Summer's explosion of energy is easily seen in our gardens. Flowers seem to grow inches overnight while vegetables go from tiny shoots to fully-formed plants in a matter of days. The bees are everywhere, with butterflies helping pollinate flowers in a haphazard way. For many of us, this is a time of staying out of nature's way while we try to keep cool.

Now is the time for capturing the flavors of our gardens—summer's bounty—to enjoy all through the year.

Herbal Vinegars

Flavored vinegar is one of the easiest ways to bring the zest of summer into otherwise dull foods. These recipes benefit from good-quality vinegar with an acetic content of 5 percent or more. Straining the vinegar after its initial flavoring will preserve its clarity and shelf life (strained, it will last up to 12 months; unstrained, it is more like 4 months). Always seal with noncorrosive lids or corks. Keep away from warmth (it can ferment) and make sure you seal it well to keep the liquid from evaporating.

Blueberry-Basil Vinegar

Here in the Pacific Northwest, the blueberry season is brief but abundant. I love making this vinegar for gifts. A dash on my winter salad greens never fails to evokes memories of the glorious summer for me.

1   large bunch of basil, washed and shaken dry

1   pound blueberries, washed and de-stemmed

4   cups white wine vinegar

Strip basil leaves from stems and tear into small pieces (about 1-inch squares). Place blueberries and 1 cup of vinegar into a nonmetallic bowl. Using the back of a wooden spoon, crush the berries to release their juices. Stir in the remaining vinegar and the basil. Pour into a large sterilized jar. Seal and shake well. Keep in a cool dark place for about 4 weeks, shaking the jar every 2 to 3 days.

Strain the vinegar through a double layer of cheesecloth into sterilized bottles to within ⅛ inch of top. Seal and label. Makes about 3⅔ cups.

Herbes de Provence Vinegar

4 sprigs each of fresh rosemary, tarragon, thyme

6 fresh bay leaves

2 pinches of fennel seeds

4 cups red wine vinegar

Lightly bruise the fresh herbs and put into a large sterilized jar with the fennel seeds. Pour in vinegar. Seal and shake well. Keep in a cool dark place for about 3 weeks, shaking the jar every 2 to 3 days. Strain the vinegar through a double layer of cheesecloth into sterilized bottles to within ⅛ inch of top. Seal and label. Makes about 1 quart.

Preserves

Each year, I make batches of preserves for my family and friends. Sweet and savory, they please everyone.

Blueberry-Lemon Jam

Some years I've "botched" this jam and it didn't set up quite right. However, it's too tasty to throw away, so I labeled it a sauce—perfect for pancakes or ice cream—and everyone liked it just as much.

1 lemon, peeled, seeded and finely chopped

1½ pints frozen-fresh blueberries

3 cups sugar

½ cup water

Place all ingredients in a large saucepan and bring to a boil, stirring constantly until blueberries pop and sugar dissolves.

Boil gently, uncovered, stirring occasionally until thickened, usually about 30 minutes. Pour into hot sterilized ½-pint jars. Process in boiling water bath for 10 minutes. Yield: 1½ pints.

Stone Fruit Chutney

This recipe is perfect for my friends who can't have sugar. Served with meat (especially pork, but not fish) or strong cheeses, this can be an elegant addition to a meal . . . or it can be a condiment slathered on a sandwich.

4 apricots

3 peaches

2 nectarines

4 plums

½ teaspoon cinnamon

2 teaspoons garlic, minced

2 teaspoons ginger, minced

1 teaspoon salt

½ teaspoon white pepper

¼ cup cider vinegar

Peel all fruit and cut into medium-sized chunks. Bring to a boil in a saucepan and cook, stirring often until the fruit is tender (15 minutes). Lower heat, add spices, and heat for 1 minute.

Boil over medium-high heat for about 45 minutes or until thick, stirring frequently. Ladle chutney into hot, sterilized, preserving jars, leaving ½ inch of space below the rim. Wipe rims clean. Seal according to manufacturer's directions. Process for 15 minutes in a boiling water bath. After processing, allow chutney to age for at least one month before using. Yield: 6 half-pint jars.

Autumn

Autumn gently leads us into the quiet time of the year. Our gardens have been harvested, flowers gently pruned and covered for their sleep, vegetable plants plowed under to fertilize the soil. This is the time for us to recover from the frantic pace of summer's bounty, to put up what we canned, and to enjoy the quiet before the holidays are upon us.

Dream Pillows

Raw Materials Needed: Two 5 × 5-inch squares of close-woven fabric of your choice, muslin bag for herbs, button, a silk cord, and filling (see below).

Sew the two pieces together along three sides, wrong side of the fabric on the outside. Turn right-side out (you now have a "bag.") Now sew the button to the outside of one side of the opening. On the inside of the opposite side, sew the silk cord in a loop. This will hold the opening closed when the herbs are inside.

Fill the muslin bag with the herbal filling and place inside the cover. Close button and place on the bed. Note: this pillow is for scent, not to actually lay your head on.

For the Filling:

- ¼ cup each of dried lemon verbena, rose petals, chamomile, rosemary or lavender
- 15 drops rose or lavender essential oil
- ¼ cup large pieces of orrisroot
- 1 cup dried hops flowers

A week before sewing the pillow, mix all of the ingredients except the hops together into a quart jar, orrisroot on top. Sprinkle oil on the orrisroot. Shake every day. Just before placing in pillow, add hops.

Alternative filling ingredients: catnip, lemon balm, marjoram, and/or sweet woodruff. Alternative essential oils: hyacinth, jasmine, lilac; and/or peppermint.

Rosemary Hair Rinse

During the winter, many of us suffer from dry scalp because of the dry heat of our homes. To combat this, I use a hair rinse that is made from the last of the rosemary in my garden.

2 handfuls of fresh rosemary stems

2 jars with plastic screw-top lids

1 pint white vinegar

1 pint water

Nonreactive saucepan

Coffee filter

Wash the rosemary gently in very cold water and shake dry. Break into 2- to 3-inch lengths and divide equally between the jars. In the saucepan, bring water and vinegar to a gentle boil. Remove from heat and let stand for 2 minutes. Pour the hot water and vinegar mixture equally over rosemary.

Seal the jars and let stand in a warm, sun-filled place for 2 weeks. Shake every 3 days. Strain decoction through the coffee filter into new bottles.

To use: massage into the scalp after washing hair. Leave in for best effect. If the smell is too intense, leave in for 30 minutes and then rinse with lukewarm water.

The garden provides many items to make wonderful, unusual, and practical crafts. May you enjoy its creative bounty all through the year!

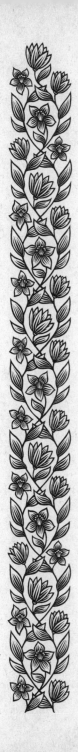

Herb
History,
Myth, and
Lore

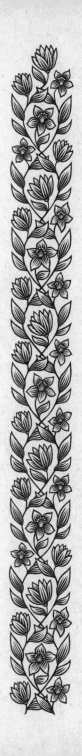

Nightshades and the Notorious

❧ by Magenta Griffith ❧

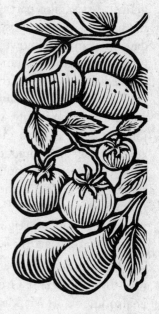

Most herbs are useful for food, medicine, or cosmetics—sometimes all of these. But there are a few that are quite dangerous—perhaps useful in small, precise doses for certain ailments, but otherwise poisonous—and to be avoided. That said, some of the most dangerous plants are also the most intriguing. Take the nightshades, which refers to both the family Solanaceae. The botanical family is large and includes ordinary plants like potatoes, tomatoes, eggplants, chili peppers, and petunias. Tobacco is also in the nightshade family; nicotine, the main alkaloid in tobacco, is a deadly poison and is used as an insecticide. Tomatoes were once thought to be poisonous because they are members of the nightshade family, and the original small tomatoes resemble nightshade berries. Some people are allergic to all of the nightshades, and it is thought that eating any nightshade vegetable, like potatoes, will make arthritis worse.

The genus *Solanum* is a smaller category. These plants are characterized by white or purplish star-shaped flowers and usually have orange or red berries. One of the best known is the **black nightshade** (*Solanum niger*), which was named for the unusual dull, black color of its berries. Native to Europe, it has spread throughout the United States, where it is now one of the most common species of Solanum found growing wild. Because its leaves are poisonous, it is sometimes called deadly nightshade in America. Touching it can irritate the skin, and it should not be eaten by people or pets.

In Europe, deadly nightshade usually refers to **belladonna** (*Atropa belladonna*), which is very dangerous. Every part of the belladonna plant is extremely poisonous. Do not handle leaves or berries if there are any cuts or abrasions on your hands, and wash your hands after touching any part of the plant. The belladonna genus, *Atropa*, also part of the family Solanaceae, is named after the Greek Fate, Atropos, who cut the thread of life. In Chaucer's day, the plant was known as 'Dwale,' which was probably derived from the Scandinavian *dool*, meaning "sleep." Others have derived the word from the French *deuil* (grief), a reference to its fatal properties. *Belladonna* means "beautiful lady" in Italian. In sixteenth century Italy, women would put drops of belladonna juice in their eyes to give them a wide-eyed, dreamy appearance—a very risky practice just to be more attractive. Belladonna is deadly because it contains atropine, which eye doctors use in minuscule amounts in the drops to dilate the pupils. It also affects the nervous system and stimulates the heart. Injections of atropine at the proper dosage can be used to treat extremely low heart rate and cardiac arrest; larger amounts are deadly.

Mandrake, another species of *Atropa* (*A. Mandragora*), was used by the ancient Greeks as an anesthetic for operations. It is also known as Mandragora, Circe's plant, and Bryony roots.

Mandrake has long been considered a panacea, a cure-all, because the three- to four-foot long root is roughly shaped like a person's body, with a torso, four limbs, and a knob for a head.

It was thought that when the root was pulled from the earth, it would emit a scream. Supposedly, this shriek could madden, deafen, or even kill an unprotected human; the occult literature includes complex directions for harvesting a mandrake root in relative safety. This involved digging a groove around the root until its lower part was exposed, then tying a dog to it. Then the person would retreat to a safe distance and call the dog. The dog would respond, and pull up the root; thus, the dog would die instead of the person harvesting the plant. After this, the root could be safely picked off the ground. Legend has it that mandrake increases fertility in women, but this is an understudied subject. Due to the presence of atropine, it is also quite poisonous.

Jimsonweed (*Datura stramonium*), also known as thornapple, is another member of the nightshade family. No one is sure if it originated in North America or Europe. It has jagged leaves and white, trumpet-shaped flowers. The seed capsules are green, about the size of a walnut and covered with numerous sharp spines, which is probably the origin of the plant's name. The whole plant is poisonous, but the seeds are the most dangerous; neither drying nor boiling destroys the poison. The usual results of ingesting this plant are dilation of the pupil with corresponding loss of focus (and sometimes sight), giddiness, delirium, and even mania. The amount for a fatal dose varies greatly. The alkaloid consists chiefly of hyoscyamine, associated with atropine and hyoscine (scopolamine). The Tarahumara of Chihuahua, Mexico, believe jimsonweed originated in the lowermost region of the universe—a hellish place complete with a devil and other malevolent beings. Legend holds that jimsonweed can cast a powerful spell on an unsuspecting forager and only people of great spiritual authority, such as a renowned shaman, can collect this plant without rousing its dangerous spirits.

Monkshood (*Aconitum napellus*), also known as wolfbane, is about three feet high, with dark green, glossy divided leaves, and flowers in erect clusters of a dark blue color. The shape of the flower is likely to attract bees. The sepals are purple—which is especially attractive to bees—and are fancifully shaped, one of them being in the form of a hood, hence the name. The roots are extremely poisonous, but all parts of the plant are dangerous. Aconite has been a well-known poison since ancient times and is derived from plants in the *Aconitum* genus. Aconite can cause death by respiratory and heart failure. However, it can also relieve pain and inflammation, dilate blood vessels, and act as an anesthetic. It is used in homeopathy and traditional Chinese herbal medicine.

Henbane (*Hyoscyamus niger*) is another deadly European plant. The medicinal uses of henbane date from the first century AD to produce sleep and ease pain. The leaves, the seeds, and the juice cause a restless sleep when taken internally, said to be "like unto the sleep of drunkenness, which continueth long and is deadly to the patient." Some thought washing the feet in a decoction of henbane or smelling the flowers would cause sleep. All parts of the plant contain scopolamine, atropine, and hyoscyamine and are therefore dangerous; neither drying nor boiling destroys the poison. In some folklore, necklaces were made from the root and were hung about the necks of children as charms to prevent fits and to cause easy teething. In Shakespeare's play *Hamlet*, the ghost of Hamlet's father reveals to his son that he was murdered when a distillation of henbane was poured in his ear.

The Notorious

Other plants besides the nightshades are infamous because of their deadly properties. **Hemlock** (*Conium maculatum*) has been a known poison for thousands of years. The plant's notoriety comes from its use in the execution of the famous Greek philosopher, Socrates, who was forced to drink an extract from the plant. The most lethal compound found in hemlock is coniine, a neurotoxin that disrupts the central nervous system. However, hemlock also has sedative and antispasmodic properties, which is why Greek and Arab physicians used it to treat arthritis and other problems. But the difference between a therapeutic dose and a toxic dose is very small, and overdoses can cause paralysis, loss of speech, difficulty breathing, and death. Although not native to the United States, it has become established here and is a fairly common roadside weed. It can grow up to ten feet tall and is easily recognized by the purple splotches on its stem. Contact with this plant can cause skin irritation. (The hemlock tree is not poisonous.)

Foxglove (*Digitalis purpurea*) is a beautiful plant that grows up to three feet tall with drooping purple, pink, or white flowers. But because just a nibble of the plant's leaves can be enough to cause death, it has sinister nicknames, including "Dead Man's Bells" and "Witches' Gloves." If you eat any part of these plants in the wild, you will likely have heart problems after a spell of nausea, vomiting, cramps, diarrhea, and pain in the mouth. Other names for this plant include fairy bells, rabbit flower, throatwort, and Witches' thimbles. Digotoxin is extracted from this plant. However, the same toxin that is deadly can be used to treat heart conditions. Digotoxin is useful for treating atrial fibrillation, atrial flutter, and as a last resort medication for congestive heart failure.

Every bit of the **oleander** plant (*Nerium oleander*), found in the southern United States and tropics, is extremely toxic. People have become very ill from merely using the sticks for roasting hot dogs or marshmallows. Even burning this bush creates a deadly smoke, and anyone who ingests its leaves, flowers, or stems can suffer sever gastric disturbances, breathing problems, comas, and death. Oleander contains a cardiac glycoside similar to that found in foxglove. Typically the symptoms involve a change in heart rate (sometimes slowing down, sometimes palpitating) or high potassium levels.

Rhododendron and **azaleas** are beautiful ornamental shrubs. However, the plants are so poisonous even the honey from bees that gathered nectar from its flowers can be toxic. This has been used as a tactic in warfare. Xenophon, a brilliant military leader and a follower of Socrates, found out the hard way. In 401 BC, following a less-than-optimal campaign in Persia, he led ten thousand Greek soldiers through the mountains of Kurdistan, Georgia, and finally Armenia. They noticed a large number of beehives when they made camp in Colchis. They raided the hives and devoured the honey. Soon they were all acting like intoxicated madmen, had fits of vomiting, and collapsed by the thousands. Pompey camped in the same area in 67 BC while campaigning against Mithridates, king of Pontus. Some allies of Mithridates had placed toxic honeycombs all along the way. Pompey's army feasted on the honeycombs and soon they were easily slaughtered. This honey became known as *meli maenomenon*, Latin for "mad honey." Similar tactics were used against Russian foes of Olga of Kiev in AD 946, and Tartar soldiers were massacred by the Russians in 1489.

Today in the United States, poison control databases all mention toxic honey poisoning. The toxin produced in the nectar of the poisonous rhododendron species varies greatly. Early symptoms include tingling, numbness, dizziness, and impaired speech. Larger amounts result in vertigo, delirium, nausea and vomiting, impaired breathing, low blood pressure, muscle paralysis, and unconsciousness. The bees are not immune, by the way.

Though usually useful, a few herbs are deadly. A useful website is the Cornell University Poisonous Plants Informational database, www.ansci.cornell.edu/plants/comlist.html, which the animal husbandry department sponsors because so many of these plants are dangerous to grazing animals. It's also useful for gardeners.

The historical association of nightshades with poison and death is so strong that a publisher of horror and dark fantasy novels took the name Nightshade Books. Better to read about them than to taste them!

Plants of the Bible

≈ by Cheryl Hoard ≈

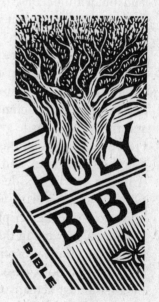

The story of the plants of Biblical lands is better understood when we appreciate what a significant region this has been since before the earliest written record. This area, known as the Fertile Crescent, is the meeting point of the African, Asian, and European continents and has commanded a huge role in the development of the modern world. What makes this even more remarkable is how small the Bible lands were. What we know today as the Syria-Lebanon-Jordan-Palestine-Egypt-Sinai region is roughly the size of New York and Maryland. There may be no other land area on Earth of this small size that offers the variety of climates and phytogeography that the Biblical lands offer. Compare the snow-capped mountains 10,000 feet high near Teheran to the Dead Sea, which is 1,292 feet below sea level.

In between, there are tropics, lush meadows, coastal regions, sand dunes, deserts and, last but not least, the fertile Nile River delta and valley. This huge variety of climates and geography contributed to the early success of inhabitants of this land developing crops and animal husbandry.

With such a range in growing conditions and vegetation, it's no wonder that no other botanical topic has been explored in this extreme detail by so many scholars and for so many centuries as the plants of the Bible. Unfortunately, the names of plants mentioned in modern translations are not as accurate as we might assume. The original writers of the Bible were not botanists or natural historians. Botany as a science wasn't developed until much later in history and the writers of the Scriptures were focused upon other concepts involving morality and theology. These ancient authors were certainly keenly interested in the plants of their land, but without consistent botanical nomenclature in place (and further clouded by translations), despite exhaustive discussion and debate, their reports were not reliable.

As translations were written and the Bible was first distributed to many different countries, translators did not realize that the same plants were not present in all countries of the world due to variations in climate, altitude, and soil content. Scholars and theologians made great efforts to discover the origin of the Hebrew plant name, then searched their homelands of France, Germany, England, and other countries of Europe and North America for plants described by ancient writers of Rome, Greece, and Arabia. Even more amusing to us today is their effort to scour the Scriptures attempting to find descriptions of the plants growing in their northern countries. Needless to say, finding a definitive profile of plants from that era is difficult. In fact, the first book based on the observations of Biblical plants by a naturalist actually exploring the Holy Land was not published until 1757. Even then, scholars and museum visitors were already noting the relative wealth of natural history information about the rest of the world—including the most remote parts of India—when compared to the Bible lands.

Even after most people realized that lands contained their own unique groups of native plants, identifying Biblical plants was still complicated because of changes over time. Many native plants had already disappeared or dwindled to small traces in the Holy Land because of environmental changes due to overcultivation and destruction of forests. As far back as 700 BC, the land has suffered not only from natives using the resources, but also from repeated invasions resulting in many more populations occupying this small area. This can be better appreciated when you compare three thousand to four thousand years of cultivation on the Bible land to how much the United States has changed in the last three hundred years due to an expanding population and cultivation. Today, plants from all over the world grow in these areas, but only some of the original plants are still evident. Parts of the Holy Land, once called the land of milk and honey, used to be rife with date palms and cedars—species that now must be carefully cultivated and protected by various governments.

Fiction or Fact?

Some may be disappointed to learn that hyssop, calamus, rose, lily, blue vervain, elm, sycamore, chestnut, and willow are plants of European and American countries. These did not grow in Biblical lands in ancient times. It's not uncommon to see paintings of Biblical figures with recently introduced plants such as cacti in the background. Cactus is a plant native to the Americas and definitely did not grow in Biblical areas until quite recently.

It's important to realize that some material in the Old Testament was actually poetry, folksongs, and ballads passed on for generations in the oral tradition for many hundreds of years. Because much of this material predates any written language, parts of the Bible could have originated as early as 4000 BC. Furthermore, this information was not documented all at once.

Some sections of the Old Testament were written by 400 BC with other parts continuing to be completed by the tenth century AD. With many scribes contributing, inconsistencies in the overall document were inevitable. However, there were also discrepancies within individual stories. The transcribing of some oral tales were often started by one scribe and finished by others. The lack of clarity in plant terminology is understandable.

The many translations have contributed to the problem as well. The Hebrew Bible was first translated into Greek between the third and first centuries BC, but the oldest Hebrew text now known to us is thought to have been written between the eighth and tenth centuries AD. The Authorized Version of King James, completed in 1611, has greatly perpetuated the botanical confusion because of the popularity and wide distribution of this English translation. Sadly, botany was not fully developed at this time in history.

Despite the confusion, some aromatic medicinal plants that were definitely present or in significant use at this time include cassia, cinnamon, galbanum, frankincense, myrrh, and spikenard. Aromatics and herbs have played a large influential role in health, healing, religion, lifestyle, and business since the beginning of recorded history. They were imported and exported between the three continents of Asia, Africa, and Europe during Biblical times. Just the pursuit and trade in these exotics alone changed the destinies of nations and civilizations. They were used for medicine, sacrificial or religious items, cosmetics, embalming, and in place of currency to buy commodities or services. Eventually, trade opened up between Eastern and Western countries facilitating cultural exchange of religion and lifestyle and also leading to the discovery of new lands, including the Americas.

Trade in these precious aromatics was big business. While some aromatics were abundant and relatively easy to harvest, the long and difficult transport to the neighboring countries made them expensive. The oldest known trade route was thought to be 2,400 miles long. Nonetheless, the Spice Kingdom vigorously thrived from 1500 to 500 BC in aromatics and spices from the Far East; gold, pearls and precious stones from India; and ivory and myrrh from East Africa. Arabia greatly prospered from 2000 BC up to the first century AD by transporting these valuable goods to other countries. Frankincense, one of Arabia's most valuable domestic products, was in great demand as incense and was carried along what was known as the "incense route" to the markets of Egypt, Persia, Babylon, Assyria, Greece, and Rome. Geographically, the Arabians were in the middle between the buyers and suppliers of these precious items. As middlemen, they easily had quite a monopoly on these exotics. The Greek influence extended to many areas during the last few centuries BC. After Alexander the Great conquered Egypt, the Greek trade route eventually became known as the "Silk Road."

Traditional, Ritual Uses

Today just a few hundred tons of frankincense is produced annually, but in the heyday of incense aromatics around 300 BC, about 3,000 tons of frankincense alone was exported. At that time, a Greek historian and traveler recorded that 1,000 talents (about 98,422 pounds) was the annual tribute given to the Babylonian King Nebuchadnezzar for ceremonial use in the great temple of Baal. The immense quantities of these aromatics produced, traded, and stockpiled during this time of history also show just how profuse their use was at ancient burials. Bodies were anointed and embalmed while aromatics were wrapped within burial clothes. The Romans were the most avid users of aromatics. In AD 66, as a measure of his grief, the emperor Nero is said to have burned a year's supply of Rome's cinnamon during his wife's funeral rites as well as more incense (probably frankincense) than Arabia could produce in ten years. Another factor that is considered credible is that perhaps huge amounts of these highly pungent and fragrant substances were actually needed in these warm climates so that mourners could be near the deceased and participate in the burial rites.

Regardless of weather, pleasant fragrance was clearly valued during biblical days as evidenced by the numerous mentions of uses for aromatic spices and resins in the Bible. Unpleasant odors were thought to be evil, but clean, beautiful scents were associated with purity and goodness. From this belief, a demand was established for these aromatics to be used ceremoniously to please the ancient gods and banish evil spirits, insects, and pests. The Dead Sea Scrolls stated that on the Sabbath, every person should wash their clothes and then rub them with frankincense. Every Sabbath day, the holy bread was placed on the altar along with frankincense in the tabernacle. The rising smoke of incense was thought to form a link between the people and their gods in heaven. Incense was burned for several reasons: as a sacrifice to god, sacrifice to a dead person, to honor a living person, for the forgiveness of sins, to ward off evil spirits, and as a pleasant or festive fragrance at banquets and events. Illness was thought to be caused by evil spirits.

Historical, Present-Day Medicinal Uses

Starting around 4000 BC, nearly all the ancient records concerning medicine, perfume, and incense from many countries mentioned in the Bible books included frankincense and myrrh. The gum resins collected from these small, unimpressive, shrublike trees and other aromatic parts of other plants were sometimes soaked or infused in animal or vegetable fat. The fat acted as a solvent and extracted many of the natural, medicinal constituents of the plant material, including the scent. Ointments or salves were made utilizing this method as well as unguent cones, which were placed on top of a person's head as depicted on the walls of tombs and temples. The heat of the day caused the cone to slowly melt down over the hair and upper body. Essential oils, produced by distillation, of these same aromatics are in popular use today, but there is no evidence that distillation took place on a scale that would have allowed for essential oils to be in use during these ancient times. Regrettably, aromatherapy authors often refer to essential oil use during the Egyptian, Greek, and Roman eras. Undoubtedly, the ointments and ungents were skillfully made so strong that their aromas were certainly therapeutic. Here is a closer look at a few well-known Bible plants that are still widely used today.

Frankincense (*Boswellia carteri*) salves and plasters were used to heal sores or wounds, and many cosmetic products were made including a hair lacquer from fresh frankincense gum to hold elaborate hair styles in place. For broken limbs, the soft gum of frankincense was placed between layers of bark that molded to the shape of the limb when the resin hardened. The bark and resin were boiled and taken as tea for fevers, tumors, gastrointestinal problems, syphilis, urinary infections, and as an antidote for arrow poison. As an aid during pregnancy, it helped morning sickness, eased labor, and promoted healing and recovery after birth. Today, frankincense is highly regarded for respiratory complaints, especially because of its bronchodilation ability, strong infection-fighting action, and as a soothing agent for coughs. In Traditional Chinese Medicine, the pills and tea are used for menstrual pain, skin problems, leprosy, and cancer. In more parts of the world today, the alcohol extract is showing great promise as an anti-inflammatory for arthritis. Many ancient aromatics, including frankincense, were used for embalming. Plants that preserved as well as they did for this historical purpose can easily be shown to be of great value for preserving the beauty of the skin. Frankincense happens to be famous for its cell-regenerating effect, making it a premier ingredient for moisturizing lotions and facials while also explaining part of its wound-healing and scar-reduction benefit. Today the essential oil of frankincense is commonly used for colds, flu, asthma, cosmetics, and wound healing. The intensely fragrant essential oil is also greatly beneficial for its relaxing, grounding effect when inhaled. It's not hard to imagine a substance that deepens the breath would be an integral part of a religious ceremony. Frankincense was quite probably the most significant ceremonial aromatic, possibly because of this profound calming effect. The word *frankincense* means "true incense."

Myrrh (*Commiphora myrrha*) gum resin was thought to be even more medicinal than frankincense. While also used ceremoniously, it was more of a medicine compared to frankincense. A past and present cure-all for mouth and gum problems, ancient texts list it as a treatment for just about everything, including delirium, epilepsy, paralysis, fatigue, palsy, gout, coughs, constipation and dysentery. Famous for wound healing, myrrh is also a strong infection-fighting agent and cell regenerator. For women, it was considered a tonic for the uterus, helping quell problems such as fertility and menstrual irregularities and sometimes even uterine tumors. Popular modern uses include the powder, alcohol extract, and essential oil used for healing wounds, combating fungus, and stopping excess mucus in respiratory problems.

Cassia (*Cinnamomum cassia*) and **Cinnamon** (*Cinnamomum zeylanicum*), cousins from the Far East with similar scents, were some of the earliest recorded spices. Cassia is actually what America calls cinnamon, and when you buy a jar of cinnamon at the market in Britain, it is actually the true cinnamon (*C. zeylanicum*). The pursuit of cinnamon from another source besides Ceylon indirectly led to the discovery of the Americas. At the time of Biblical activity in the Fertile Crescent, cinnamon and cassia bark were used medically for the digestive and respiratory systems as well as to treat infections. Their strong beautiful aromas were revered for ceremonial use, as noted by numerous mentions in the Bible. The herb itself and the essential oils are used today to treat the same problems. Cassia powder is gaining interest after studies recently proved it can lower blood sugar. Just a half-teaspoon a day taken in the diet or in capsules is all that is needed. These essential oils are irritating to the skin and are mostly used for inhalation, mouthwashes, toothpastes, and as flavoring.

The earliest civilizations used **Galbanum** (*Ferula galbaniflua*), for incense, embalming, treating wounds and skin problems, and as medicine for many other major body systems. Galbanum is a large perennial herb from which today an oleoresin is harvested, dried, and then distilled to produce the essential oil. The essential oil is considered valuable for supporting the health of the skin as well as comforting the respiratory system and muscular/skeletal system. Its actions are skin-cell regenerating, analgesic, antiseptic, anti-inflammatory, and antispasmodic. Essential oils have quite a reputation for healing the spirit, and galbanum has been successful for calming emotional extremes by fostering a feeling of balance, which is good for nervous tension, erratic moods, and is even a treatment for hysteria and paranoia. It also aids meditation and is thought to help resolve old problems of an emotional nature.

Spikenard (*Nardostachys jatamansi*), also known as Nard, was an expensive aromatic from India that was often exported in sealed alabaster boxes and used as perfume and as a circulatory remedy. During Biblical days, when the master of the house received guests, the seal of the alabaster box would be broken and the honored guests would be anointed with this highly prized ointment. The ancient Hebrews and Romans used spikenard ceremonially to bury the dead. Today, the fragrant root of this plant, which is closely related to valerian, is distilled to produce the essential oil. Spikenard can be used to comfort the skin, but its most popular uses are inhalation for counteracting stress and anxiety and for religious purposes—even today it is applied as anointing oil.

Great benefits can be gained by incorporating these essential oils into your lifestyle. A few drops (maximum fifteen) can be added to your bath water or you can try adding a maximum of fifteen drops to an ounce of vegetable oil or aloe gel for body lotions. For face products, use only three to five drops of essential

CLINTON PUBLIC LIBRARY
CLINTON, IOWA
52732

oil in an ounce of vegetable oil. Stress may be one of biggest factors contributing to the occurrence of minor illness and major disease. The stress-reduction benefits of these historical old world aromatics is enough incentive to begin to explore their use in daily life. I feel I greatly benefit from diffusing these essential oils around my house, in aromatic baths, and using them in my body care products, soaps, and shampoos. To have an understanding of how significant these exotics have been in shaping the world as we know it today increases the appreciation of their scents. For me, their pungent, resinous scents evoke a sense of awareness of ancient Earth and give instant stabilizing comfort. Often, this occurs during rushed moments, such as when we wash our hands or put on hand lotion. When I perceive these aromas at those times it helps me to remember what is important in life.

For Further Reading

Battaglia, Salvatore. *The Complete Guide to Aromatherapy*. Virginia, Queensland: The Perfect Potion, 1995.

Diamond, Jared. *Guns, Germs, and Steel*. New York: W.W. Norton & Company, 1999.

Lawless, Julia. *The Illustrated Encyclopedia of Essential Oils*. Shaftesbury, Dorset: Element Books Limited, 1995.

Moldenke, Harold N. and Moldenke, Alma L. *Plants of the Bible*. New York: Dover Publishing, Inc., 1986.

Rosengarten, Frederic. *The Book of Spices*. New York: Pyramid Books, 1973.

Sheppard-Hanger, Sylla. *The Aromatherapy Practitioner Reference Manual, Vol. 1, Vol. 2*. Tampa: Atlantic Institute of Aromatherapy, 1997.

Resplendent Rose

⪢ by Ember ⪡

O ne of the world's most well-known and beloved flowers, the rose has a long and complex history. Valued for its beauty, folklore, and even medicinal properties, the rose can be enjoyed in a variety of ways, from cosmetics and cooking to gardening and crafts.

Our current roses have descended from wild ancestors of temperate and subtropical climates, but this lineage is difficult to trace. We do know, however, that the rose is ancient. Fossils have been found that are over 35 million years old. Today, we cultivate about three thousand varieties of this magnificent flower.

The older roses of the past had only five petals. Some of these wild natives can still be identified today. The rose as we know it is a member of a large family, Rosaceae, which contains many

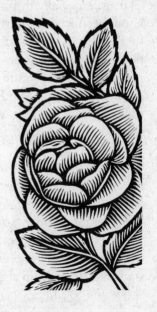

plants related to roses such as apples, strawberries, peaches, plums, apricots, raspberries, rowan, cinquefoil, blackberries, almonds, hawthorn, and pears. The Rosaceae family is an enormous plant group with members found everywhere in the world.

Roses have been revered for centuries and rose legends abound. They were used by the ancient Egyptians, Greeks, and Romans. Rumor had it that the floors of Cleopatra's palace were carpeted with rose petals, and they are reputed to have been sacred to the Druids. Another interesting historical note is that early Christians rejected roses because they associated the flower with Roman debauchery. But such a lovely flower proved to be too irresistible, and eventually they, too, adopted the rose as a sacred symbol by the fifth and sixth centuries. By the thirteenth century, the rose was firmly established in Christian lore. The Catholic rosary may have received its name from the rose. One legend says that the rosary was created when the prayers of a monk changed into roses as they fell from his lips. Yet another legend claims the rose was named by Venus for her son Eros.

The rose has long been associated with love magic and charms, especially in Europe. An ancient charm for a maiden to know her future required that she gather the following on the first of July: a sprig of rosemary, a white rose, a red rose, a blue flower, a yellow flower, nine blades of long grass, and a sprig of rue. This bundle was then tied together with a lock of her hair, sprinkled with salt, and placed beneath her pillow. She would then have dreams that would reveal her future. Roses were considered to bring good fortune unless the petals fell off when it was picked.

Roses have often been used to silently or secretly communicate emotions. This started in Victorian times, and the meanings vary according to the source. Here is one traditional list: Dark red is for love, desire, and courage; dark pink expresses gratitude, appreciation, or respect; light pink is for admiration or sympathy; white is for reverence, purity, and innocence; and yellow stands for friendship and joy.

Of the great deal of healing folklore associated with roses, much is superstition, but some is based on real chemical properties. For example, we know today that rose hips, the "fruit" of the rose, contain more vitamin C than oranges and they are used in many herbal teas and remedies. The traditional rose used for medicinal purposes is *R. gallica officinalis*. One of the most popular uses is making rose water.

Rose oil and rose water are used today in cosmetics, aromatherapy, perfume, soaps, and even cooking, baking, and making tea. Rose oil is found in rose petals and is often called attar or otto. The oil is very precious—it takes sixty thousand roses to make one ounce—which is why it's so expensive!

You can purchase rose water from specialty shops or make your own at home to use in cooking or as a face wash. But be sure you use organic roses; never consume rose water made with plants treated with chemicals or pesticides. Freshly picked organic petals from your own garden work the best. Sometimes florists can get organic roses for you if you ask.

To make rose water, put two cups of firmly packed petals and two and one-fourth cups of water in a saucepan and simmer, covered, over low heat until the water is reduced by half. Cool. Strain out the petals and store in a sterile jar or bottle out of direct sunlight. Another method is to just put the petals in a glass bowl and pour boiling water over them. Then cover and let them sit for twenty to thirty minutes, and then strain. Rose water won't keep long, perhaps up to ten days in the refrigerator, unless you add alcohol as a preservative. If you add a tablespoon of vodka, it will last about a month. Used in a spray bottle, it makes a nice air-freshening mist or tonic for the skin.

Another fun way to enjoy roses is by eating candied rose petals or using them for decorations on a cake. First, pinch off the white tip of each petal, since this part tastes bitter. Whisk one egg white with a tablespoon of water and dip each petal in the mix or brush petal with mixture. Drain them on wax paper and, while still damp, sprinkle petals with granulated sugar on both sides. Shake off the excess and place them back on wax paper to dry for at least twelve hours. Store covered, in the refrigerator. They'll keep for about one month.

And finally, if you grow roses or have been given a lovely bouquet, you can dry them to make arrangements and wreaths. Working with dried roses is easy as long as you handle them with care. Hang the roses upside down away from direct sunlight and drafts. In about a week, they will be brittle—extremely fragile! When they're dry, simply put them in a vase or carefully cut off the stems and use a hot glue gun to attach the blossoms to a grapevine wreath. If desired, you can spray them with a preservative (available at most craft stores). Add other dried flowers or herbs to the wreath and decorate it with ribbons.

There are many ways to experience roses beyond the garden or vase. However you choose to enjoy them, you're in good company with those whose lives have been touched by the rose throughout history. The rose is truly a queen among flowers.

Herbs of the Southwest

≫ by Kristin Madden ≪

A group of Paleolithic hunters roams farther than ever before, searching in vain for the large animals they depend on. Desperation, observation, and the guidance of their gods leads them to experiment with the plants that remain in their world. From this time forward, these people and their descendants will discover food, medicines, clothes, tools, and ceremonial items among the flora of the Earth and cultures will be forever changed.

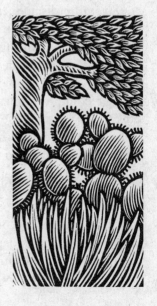

With the mass extinctions that occurred around 6000 BC, the peoples of the Southwestern United States had one choice: find another means of subsistence or die. As a result, herbs and other plants became an integral part of Native American culture in the southwest. When the Spanish arrived with their *curanderas* (women who practice folk medicine) and traditions, another layer of herbal lore was laid upon the rich history of the Southwest. Medicinal and edible plants have been wildcrafted and cultivated in this region for many thousands of years.

What Did Early People Use?

Legends offer us our first insights into the lives of early peoples. Myths, ancient stories, and folklore all provide clues for us to follow. Whether literal or symbolic, these stories developed from something meaningful to our ancestors. The fact that they have survived the centuries may mean only that they are great stories. But it may also mean that this information struck a chord within each succeeding generation . . . a remaining thread of a truth long forgotten that we are not prepared to let go of completely.

Folklore often offers modern people the best clues. Traditional healer methods and "old wives' tales" are handed down from generation to generation. Many of these ancient tales are so worth exploring that large pharmaceutical companies have been sending ethnobotanists into areas like the Southwest for decades in the hopes of "discovering" a new miracle drug.

Scientific disciplines have developed to allow us to follow these threads into the past. Archeology is perhaps the most obvious. Rock paintings and carvings, village sites, and food containers provide clues to daily life. Palynology (the study of pollen), dendrochronology (the study of tree rings), and carbon-dating techniques allow us to identify the plants found in ancient sites and place their use within a fairly specific time frame. And archeobotany helps us intepret the plant parts found in prehistoric sites in relation to the people who used them.

Natural First Aid

Have you ever used jojoba oil lip balm for chapped lips? Or aspirin for pain or as a blood thinner? Does your favorite decongestant contain pseudoephedrine? These fairly common first-aid remedies originated with plants of the Southwest. But there are some Southwestern powerhouses that are not as well known.

Agave (*Agave spp.*) or mescal, was once cultivated on prehistoric terraces in southwestern New Mexico. This herb is probably best known for its role in the production of tequila, made from roasted and fermented agave plants. Certainly, there are times when a shot of tequila seems like just the first aid you need, but agave itself offers much more. Tinctures and teas of agave leaf can have a laxative and relaxing effect, easing both constipation and colic. The root tincture has been shown to alleviate arthritic symptoms, but should not be used as a long-term cure for arthritis.

Jojoba (*Simmondsia chinensis*) oil is commonly found in natural lip balms and moisturizers, possibly due to its anti-inflammatory effects on mucous membranes. Teas made from jojoba leaves will ease the pain of chapped lips, fever blisters, hemorrhoids, colitis, and more. This same tea has been used in Mexico to treat asthma and emphysema. A poultice of fresh leaves will reduce inflammation of cuts, scrapes, and rashes. In a mouthwash, the leaves ease cold sores, gum disease, and sore throats. Sore throats are also aided by drinking a tea made of jojoba seeds. Teas made from jojoba leaves can relieve diarrhea and painful urination.

Juniper (*Juniperus spp.*) berries were eaten regularly by the ancestors of the Pueblo peoples and are known to stimulate digestion if chewed about an hour before eating. According to Southwestern folklore, drinking five berries each day (steeped in tea) will act as a contraceptive. Used for dyes by the Navajo, necklaces by the Hopi, and everyday tools like cordage, bows, cradles, and even toilet paper by many Pueblos, juniper has a rich history in the Southwest.

Both the berries and leaves, in teas, will aid inflammations of the urinary tract, though the tea is easier on the stomach and more effective if combined with other beneficial plants. Teas made from leaf sprigs aid in treating colds, stomach disorders, constipation, rheumatism, headaches, and nausea. This leaf-sprig tea is known to most of the Pueblo peoples of the Southwest as an important aid during labor and delivery. Juniper bark, powdered or boiled, has been known to soothe spider bites and earache.

One note of caution: juniper berries and leaves should not be using during pregnancy or by anyone with kidney problems.

Mesquite (*Prosopis spp.*) is a common shrub of the Southwest. Sometimes referred to as an indicator plant—showing where oil reserves may lie—mesquite beans were used to supplement shrinking food stores in the late 1500s by native Mexicans that accompanied some Spanish colonial trips into the desert Southwest.

While commonly used to smoke meats and add flavor to barbecues, mesquite is also widely used for medicinal purposes, largely for its astringent and antimicrobial properties. All parts of the shrub above the roots are used in teas. Even the resin that seeps out from beneath the bark is used to produce a thin, slimy paste that is a potent tool in fighting laryngitis, sore throats, and ulcers. The pods are soaked and steeped to produce a soothing eyewash for conjunctivitis and pink eye. Used in conjunction with prickly pear, mesquite tea is a wonderful wash for disinfecting cuts and soothing bruises.

Mormon Tea (*Ephedra spp.*) or 'Joint-Fir,' is a good-sized but spindly shrub that is reputed to be a powerful antidote to dehydration. Drinking the tea or chewing on the stems will stave off thirst, even on hot desert days. Found in many archeological sites, this plant clearly has a long history of use in this area. The name, Mormon Tea, is said to have originated with the Mormon taboo on drinking caffeinated beverages. Apparently, this was an acceptable alternative boost for low energy.

Mormon Tea is a nice plant for the alternative health practitioner, particularly since it does not contain the potentially dangerous chemical ephedrine. It does contain pseudoephedrine, however, and is a fantastic decongestant. Teas made from the leaves and stems have been used as a cough medicine and as a soothing lotion for dry and itchy skin. It is also moderately diuretic and commonly used for urinary disorders.

Osha (*Ligusticum porteri*) is commonly known as bear root or porter's lovage, and it is powerful medicine. The literature will give some diverse elevations for this plant, anywhere from six thousand to over ten thousand feet, but I have always known it to be mountain medicine—and in many areas of the Southwest, six thousand feet doesn't necessarily qualify as a mountain. However, you must take extra care to identify this plant with 100 percent certainty before using it from the wild because of its similarity to the poisonous hemlock.

Osha root is my personal favorite for respiratory illnesses, sore throats, coughs, and laryngitis. We mix it with cherry syrup to cover the truly terrible taste and it works like magic. It is also a potent antiviral and detoxifying plant. Osha tea or tincture may be used to ease indigestion and vomiting as well as cuts and infections of the skin.

Prickly Pear (*Opuntia spp.*) is a flat, jointed herbaceous cactus that, as an emergency food and water source, can save your life in the desert. It flowers in yellow, red, and sometimes pink, bringing color and beauty to the varied habitats in which it thrives. If you have ever used **aloe vera** (*Aloe spp.*), which does grow as an introduced species in this area, then you will love the results you get from prickly pear. The pads, also known as tunas, were a staple food to most of the ancient Pueblos, and they were eaten by the Mayan people as well. The ripe tunas are prized as a source of rich dyes, particularly by the Navajo, while the Zuni people prefer to make dyes from the fruits.

Prickly pear tunas may be used to draw out toxins and are used in swelling, bruises, cuts, burns, and insect bites. They are surprisingly effective against the pain of ant bites. With anti-inflammatory and diuretic properties, the juice is often used in conjunction with antibiotics to soothe urinary tract infections and cystitis. The flowers are useful in fighting colitis, asthma, and bronchitis. The fruits are delicious, but beware of the spiny hairs if picking them fresh.

Sagebrush (*Artemisia spp.*) was used by the ancient Fremont people of the Four Corners area for nearly everything from clothing and tools to furniture and fuel. Found in archeological sites, sagebrush was obviously also a food source for ancestral Pueblos.

One of the Navajo Life Medicines, which are highly prized for their healing properties, sagebrush is considered a general stimulant and possesses antimicrobial properties. The leaf tea (or simply chewing on the leaves) is used to disinfectant as a wash, to induce vomiting, and to prevent and cure stomach and intestinal disorders, including worms and dysentery. Powdered leaves ease diaper rash and chafing as well as digestive problems, headache, colds, sore throats, fevers, and even childbirth pain. A popular cure for respiratory ailments, breathing in the steam of boiling sagebrush leaves is a potent decongestant and some Navajo have been known to smoke the leaves to ward off loneliness.

Willow (*Salix spp.*) and the sometimes similar-looking **Cottonwood** (*Populus spp.*) make up some of our favorite species out here for shade, beauty, and wood to craft everything from furniture and drums to dyes and foodstuffs. These water-loving trees are a clear indicator of water in the desert. But they are also truly effective anti-inflammatories and painkillers. In fact, the active ingredient in aspirin, salicyclic acid, is derived from the salicin chemical in willow trees. Willow bark tea is a popular cure for fever, sore throats, toothaches, and coughs. Cottonwoods have similar properties. A poultice of cottonwood leaves will soothe sore gums, toothaches, and cuts and scrapes. Cottonwood leaf tea has also been used to ease the pain of urinary complaints.

Long-term Cures

Of the 252 essential chemicals selected by the World Health Organization, 11 percent are from plant sources. And 25 percent of all prescription drugs in the United States contain plant chemicals. Until the 1930s, when synthetic chemistry began to outpace plant derivatives in pharmaceuticals, plants were a major source of long-term cures for all that ailed us. The native peoples and early Spanish settlers of the Southwestern United States knew their land well . . . and they developed many powerful cures, some of which are now being explored for their pharmaceutical potential.

Mesquite is also excellent for digestive problems and bacterial illnesses. It has also found favor as a soothing emollient for ulcers, colitis, and conjunctivitis. Mesquite supports the development of a healthy immune system and soothes upper-respiratory inflammations.

Prickly Pear juice helps balance blood sugar and has been used as a folk cure for diabetes. Studies have indicated that this folk cure may well pan out for juvenile-onset diabetes.

Puncture Vine (*Tribulus terrestris*) is known to most of us in its range as Goat Heads. It covers the ground in empty fields and backyards with rather pretty little vines and yellow flowers. But those vines carry a dangerous weapon: nasty little spiked balls that are notorious for puncturing bicycle tires and stabbing anyone with the nerve to wear something other than fully covering shoes. But the Goat Head is also powerful medicine. Studies have shown that the seeds may help stave off high cholesterol and lessen the effects of hardening of the arteries. What's more, it has a decided effect on high blood pressure and subsequently restores balance and harmony to cardiovascular processes.

Yucca (*Yucca spp.*) is one of the plants that seem to be synonymous with the desert Southwest. Its long, sharp leaves are sometimes confused with agave but yucca can occur as short, shrublike plants or taller treelike plants, such as Joshua Tree and Spanish bayonet, as well as soaptree, banana, and narrowleaf yuccas.

The roots of these plants are rich in saponins, meaning they turn into a soapy, detergent froth when mixed with water. These plants were prized by early Southwest inhabitants as soaps and shampoos, giving hair a glossy shine, increasing strength, and even preventing baldness. Yucca soap was even used to eradicate body and head lice.

Used by native peoples to treat arthritis and rheumatoid conditions, yucca has shown great promise as an anti-inflammatory to help treat prostate and ongoing urinary problems.

Sacred Herbs

Plants have been used since our earliest days for prayers, purification, and communing with the gods. When we work with plants in this way, we are connected to Earth and sky in powerful ways.

Corn (*Zea mays*) and corn pollen are particularly sacred to the Navajo and Apache peoples, though a great many Southwestern native cultures honor this plant and use it in ceremony. It is both a blessing and a prayer and may be used to delineate the ceremonial circle. Working with corn honors the spirits of the land and promotes fertility and peace.

Juniper (*Juniperus spp.*) is commonly used for healing, protection, and purification in the form of smudge mixtures, teas, and poultices. Dried berries are thrown on rocks in sweat lodges and saunas. While willow is often seen as the traditional sweat lodge material, Navajo sweathouses are more often made from juniper wood with juniper bark covering floors. Leaves are often carried for protection and other uses by traditional Pueblos.

Sagebrush is well known for its use in sacred saunas, sweat lodges, and smudge sticks. It is regularly used to induce trance, for deepening connections with spirits, and for purification.

To many, the Southwest is a land of diverse beauty, but few recognize the plethora of life that exists in this region. Mountains are certainly green, though still dry compared to coastal ranges, but it can take a practiced eye to see the life-giving fullness that exists in the deserts. Among the cacti and rattlesnakes, the pines and oaks, the sand and rivers, exists a subtle splendor that offers us medicines, food, and all that we could possibly need for a wonderful life. Even if you never set foot in the Southwest, you may be pleasantly surprised to discover that your favorite lip balm, shampoo, or painkiller could not exist without Southwestern plants.

The Floral Clock

⪼ by Susanna Reppert ⪻

T elling time with flowers goes back to the first century and Pliny the elder who devised a "Horologe of Flora." The eighteenth century Swedish botanist Carl Linnaeus, a.k.a. "The Father of Taxonomy," also observed this phenomenon in plants. He devised a clock of flowers that had such a sense of time he could watch the progress of the day by the half hour. He recorded both the opening and the closing times, faithfully noting nature's rhythms as it directed the plants. Linneaus termed the plants "equinoctial" for those that open and close rather punctually at the same hour every day.

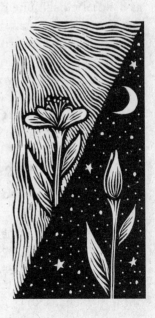

Later, they became a kind of Victorian garden game for they are listed in all the *Language of Flowers* books. The books would offer a listing of time-telling plants and encourage Victorian ladies in the pursuit of creating a parterre as a "Dial of Flowers."

In "The Floral Offering" (1868), English poet Felicity Hemans wrote:

'Twas a lovely thought to mark the hours,
as they floated in light away,
By the opening and folding flowers
That laugh to the summer's day.

Flowers that tell time have fascinated me since childhood, from the morning I chose a bunch of sparkling blue chicory as the bridal bouquet for a playground wedding. Sure enough, the flowers closed about noon, just before the performance, and the little bride, much to my chagrin, carried green stems.

The classical way to plant a floral clock is in a round flowerbed with the position of the flowers corresponding to the time on a real clock. You would need a spot that gets full sun for most of the day. Few of us would want to plant an entire garden as a floral clock. Their erratic behavior and sometimes-weedy appearances of plants would create havoc in a garden.

These plants are prone to some uncertainties, opening earlier or later depending upon the sun's intensity, temperature, and time of year—the triggers for the amazing clockworks. You may not be able to set your watch by time-telling plants, but can get a good approximation. Our garden observances have shown that fairies also use a garden of hours to gauge their days and eves.

Getting Started on Time

Here is a listing of some plants that are sure to get your botanical clock ticking.

Greeting the day at dawn is the morning glory (or wild morning glory). For the most effective and fast screen, plant the climber "heavenly blues," a stunning variety that trumpets the sun awake about 5 am to alert the fairies to return to the bottom of the garden, as it is soon time for the mortals to appear.

Around 6 am the sun gets hotter and the cape marigold opens its dark-eyed daisy flowers. By 7 am, the African marigold cheerily says "good morning world" and the white water lily greets another day.

Along about 8 am, the golden dandelion and pimpernels are willing to get up. The pimpernel goes one step further—it not only tells time but it also forecasts the weather. As "the fairies' barometer," pimpernels close for the day if rain threatens. The flower from which the Scarlet Pimpernel of fictional fame took his sobriquet is a charming little weed, popping up here and there. We always allow one to stay to tell the time and predict the weather.

By 9 am, the portulaca is in business for the day along with the bright orange calendula (winking marybuds of Shakespeare); also tawny daylilies along the roadside or in gardens and sunny hawkweed. California poppies open closer to 10 am. All brilliantly colored flowers, they seem to reflect the sun and sulk if the day be dull.

Slugabeds such as star of Bethlehem don't awaken until about 11 am, true to their French name *La Dame d'onze heures*, and the mallows herald noon. Several flowers begin their fold at noon, including morning glory (they are not called afternoon glory, for a reason) and chicory (my face still flushes at the thought of that wedding bouquet). The glorious opening of the passionflower announces lunchtime for us.

Spiderwort winds down the day at 1 pm and scarlet pimpernel has had enough of the heat by 2 pm, while at 3 pm the marigolds have closed up shop for the day.

The lucky four-o-clocks call the Wee Folk to afternoon tea at 4 pm by opening their pretty trumpet-shaped flowers.

Evening primrose, appropriately named and the state flower of Missouri, shuns the day, by waking about 6 pm and snapping shut at dawn; it is a favorite floral timepiece for the fairies—announcing both the beginning and the end of nightly festivities. Honeysuckle also opens in the evening to calm the night air with its fragrance.

By 8 pm, dandelions and daylilies have had a long day and fold their flowers.

The glowing nicotiana, moonflower, and datura permeate the night air with overpowering fragrances around 9 pm. All white flowered and shimmering in the moonlight on a hot midsummer's eve, they are a heady combination guaranteed to alert the most jaded spirits. Their bright flowers light the way for the fairies to dance the night away.

For night owls, you can set your alarm by the night blooming cereus, which opens about midnight, an exotic houseplant that blooms only after achieving some age.

Rhythms, Not Rigidity

Be warned that plants are like fairies and will not always perform precisely as scheduled nor do they observe daylight-saving time. And don't count on them to get you to the train on time. Despite such vagaries, they do indeed respond to natural elements—light, air, soil temperature, latitude—that trigger innate mechanisms to make telling time with flowers yet another adventure in gardening. This fun observation of rhythms of nature gives you a feeling of welcome when plants open to greet you, and a feeling of pleasant winding down when they close up for the day. Some are herbs, some are not, but all are useful if you observe their ingenious built-in timetables.

Traditional Scottish Staples

❧ by Ellen Evert Hopman ❧

Certain herbs and food plants have been staples of the Scottish household medicine chest and pantry for millennia. Others (such as oats) were introduced by the Romans or arrived later from the Americas (such as the potato). Here is a small sampling of the foods and medicines that ensured survival in the Highlands and lowlands of Caledonia.

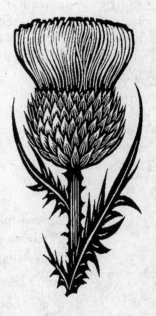

Oats

One of the plants most frequently associated with Scotland is *Avena sativa* (Gaelic – *Corc*), a household staple since Roman times. Hot oats and butter can be applied as a poultice to boils and infections. (For stubborn boils, the butter was once replaced with urine!) For coughs, colds, and fevers, a watery gruel of oatmeal is a great food.

Oatmeal is also a helpful food for colic. Flavor the gruel with butter, salt and pepper, honey, lemon, cinnamon, or raisins as desired. The ancient Celts added chopped hazelnuts and freshly chopped dandelion leaves or nettles to their oats.

To make a proper Scottish porridge, you have to use a spurtle—a wooden stirring stick that is only used for porridge. Porridge not stirred with a spurtle is not proper! Traditional porridge is cooked over low heat for about an hour with a pinch of salt, and served with butter and/or honey. (Use 1½ pints of cold water per 4 ounces of oatmeal and stir every 15 minutes.)

To treat sore eyes, soak oats in water for an hour, strain the water through a clean cloth or organic coffee filter, and apply to the eyes as a wash.

If you grow oats yourself or find them in a field, the tea of the straw is used for respiratory complaints and nervous conditions. A bath of oat straw is helpful for rheumatism, lumbago, paralysis, kidney and liver problems, gout, gravel, bladder and abdominal complaints, intestinal colic, bedwetting eczema, and shingles. A foot bath of oat straw will help tired feet. Oat straw tea can be used as a skin wash for wounds and to relieve itchy, dry skin, flaky skin conditions, sore eyes, and frostbite. To make the tea, simply simmer the straw in water for an hour and add honey if desired.

To make the bath, simmer 2 pounds of oat straw in 3 quarts of water for 30 minutes, strain, and add to the bath. Or tie a pound of oatmeal into a gauze bag and soak the bag in very hot water. Pour the water into the tub and use the gauze bag as a scrub or sponge. (Lust pp. 296–297, Beith pp. 230–231)

Scottish Oatcakes

2   cups oatmeal (use old-fashioned oats, not instant)
     Pinch sea salt
     Pinch baking soda
½   ounce beef drippings (or lard, butter)
8   ounces hot water

Mix the oatmeal, salt, and soda. Make a well in the center of the bowl, pour in the melted drippings, and then add the water until a pie-dough consistency is achieved. Cover your hands with oats and knead into a ball then roll out on a floured pastry board to ½-inch thickness. Sprinkle some oatmeal on top and cut into squares. Cook the squares on a hot griddle until the edges curl and toast slightly. (Smith-Twiddy p. 34)

Comfrey

Comfrey (*Symphytum tuberosum*) (Gaelic – *Meacan dubh*) has been introduced into American gardens, but can be found growing wild in Britain. Due to certain alkaloids present in the plant, it is best to use it externally (though homeopathic preparations of comfrey are quite dilute and safe for internal use).

A poultice of ground or mashed comfrey root and leaf can be spread on broken or fractured bones, sprains, and torn ligaments. Comfrey is a calcium precursor, which helps the body better metabolize calcium. For bone mending, chop the roots and stir them in hot water until a paste forms. Spread the paste on a clean cloth and place on the affected area for 1 hour, then discard. Repeat every 2 to 4 hours.

The powdered root and leaf are used externally to stop bleeding. Add hot water to dried comfrey or use it fresh from the garden to poultice insect bites. Cook the plant, and when soft, apply it warm to the chest for bronchitis and pleurisy.

Another method is to blend the fresh leaves with water to form a mush (or soften dried comfrey leaves with hot water). Add powdered slippery elm bark or buckwheat flour (avoid white flour, as many people are allergic to it) a little at a time until a pie dough consistency is achieved. Roll out onto a clean cloth with a rolling pin and apply to burns, wound sores, surgical scars and incisions, sores, ulcers, bruises, swelling, cuts, and fractures. (Beith, p. 212, Hopman, *A Druid's Herbal*, pp. 14–15)

Comfrey Salve

This concoction is an all-purpose skin-healing ointment for diaper rash, sunburn, kitchen burns, chafing, itchy skin, dry skin, scrapes, and dry flaky eczema.

> Comfrey leaves
>
> Horse chestnuts
>
> The green outer hull of walnuts
>
> Lavender flowers
>
> Calendula flowers
>
> Cold pressed virgin olive oil
>
> Beeswax

Fill the bottom of a large cooking pot with chopped comfrey leaves. Mix in equal parts of smashed horse chestnuts (*Aesculus hippocastanum*), which are anti-inflammatory pain relievers, using the brown shiny shell of the nut and the inner meat. Add green walnut hulls (*Juglans spp.*), which have antiseptic, antifungal, germicidal, vermicidal, and a parasiticidal qualities and also contains manganese, a skin healing agent. Fold in dried or fresh calendula flowers (*Calendula officinalis*) and lavender flowers (*Lavandula vera, L. officinalis*).

Put in enough olive oil to barely cover the plant matter (be sure to keep track of exactly how much olive oil you poured in). Cover with a tight lid and simmer for 20 minutes (do not boil).

In a separate pot, bring fresh beeswax to a simmer. When both the beeswax and the herbal mix are simmering, add 3 or 4 tablespoons of beeswax for every cup of oil you put into the pot.

While everything is still hot, strain and pour the mixture into very clean glass jars. Allow the salve to harden, then cap.

Helpful Hints: If the jars are very, very clean you won't need a preservative. Be sure to clean all utensils, pots, etc., while they are still hot to avoid hardened beeswax on your tools and pans! (Hopman, *Tree Medicine Tree Magic* pp. 115–116, 141–142, *A Druid's Herbal*, pp. 14–15)

Potato (Tatties)

Potatoes (*Solanum tuberosum*) (Gaelic – *Buntáta*) were introduced to the Highlands and the Western Isles in 1725. By 1840, 75 percent of all food consumed was potatoes. As a result, the potato famine of 1840 hit hard.

A slice of raw potato can be put over a black eye. For nosebleeds, apply raw potato slices to the back of the neck. For fevers and chest complaints, make a poultice of cooked mashed potatoes and grated fresh ginger. Apply it as hot as possible (comfortable) to the lung area to break up congestion and draw out fever.

Raw potato juice can be applied to gout, rheumatism, lumbago, sprains, bruises, and synovitis (joint inflammation). Potatoes and corn make a complete protein when eaten together.

Cut up 1 pound of unpeeled potatoes and simmer in 2 pints of water until the liquid is halved. Apply the hot water to swollen rheumatic parts.

Mash raw potato in a mortar and apply it to burns and scalds. Mash a baked potato mix in a bit of olive oil and apply it to frostbite. (Beith 234, Grieve 654–655)

Leek and Tattie Soup

1   pound potatoes, cubed

3   small leeks

1   ounce flour

1   ounce butter

2   pints stock

    Seasonings

4   ounces hard cheese

Chop the leeks, coat in flour, and fry gently in the butter. Add potatoes and the stock and season to taste. Simmer for an hour. Liquify and return to the pan. Reheat and serve with grated cheese on top. (Smith-Twiddy, p. 21). Variations of this recipe often include carrots, onions, and turnips.

Nettles

Nettles (*Urtica urens*) (Gaelic – *deanntag, feanntag*) are gathered before the plant comes into flower. I like to make a clear nettle broth (Gaelic – *cál deanntaig*) in the early spring. It is full of minerals such as iron, and also contains chlorophyll, which detoxifies the blood after a long winter. The broth is beneficial for coughs, upset stomachs, and rheumatic complaints. Nettles are warming to the system, warding off chill at the change of season.

The young greens are added to soups or cooked as a potherb. Don't be afraid of the sting; just be sure to wear good garden gloves or rubber gloves from the kitchen as you gather the plant. A quick rinse with cool water under the kitchen tap will instantly wash off the irritating acid.

The root tea is beneficial for chest complaints, and a poultice of nettles can be applied to wounds to stop bleeding. Nettle tea or juice can be ingested to stop internal bleeding. Soak a cloth in the fresh juice or the tea to stop a nose bleed. The tea is a kidney tonic (only people who are generally chilly should use it for long periods of time) and also helps diarrhea. The root tea helps kidney-centered edema.

To make nettle juice, take 1 to 2 tablespoons with an equal portion of water. To make nettle tea, steep 2 to 3 tablespoons of the leaf in 1 cup of freshly boiled water for 10 minutes.

Nettles are antihistamines that will benefit persons with allergies and hay fever. The juice of the root or leaf mixed with honey helps asthma and bronchitis. A decoction of the seeds can be added to the leaf tea to treat tuberculosis and intermittent fever. Simmer nettles with violet leaves and whey for fevers and nervous conditions. Mix the spring-gathered leaves with oatmeal to make a nourishing food for invalids. Eat nettles cooked with egg whites to promote restful sleep.

Caution: Avoid eating the old plants unless well cooked or kidney damage might occur. (Beith, p. 230, Lust, p. 291, Livingstone, p. 129)

Nettle, Onion, and Spinach Pie

1   pound young nettles

3   pounds spinach leaves (fresh or frozen)

2   onions, medium-sized

4   eggs, small

½   pound cheese, grated

     Salt and pepper

Pick the tips off the young nettles and cook them for about 10 minutes, squeeze out the liquid, and finely chop. Then do the same with the spinach leaves. Put the chopped nettle tips, spinach, and onions, into a high-sided pie dish. Beat the 4 small eggs with salt and pepper to taste, then pour the egg mixture over the vegetables. Sprinkle with ½ pound grated cheese. Cover with aluminum foil and put the dish into a container of water that comes halfway up the sides. Bake at 320 degrees F. for about 1½ hours. (Smith-Twiddy, p. 62)

Rowan – Mountain Ash

Sorbus aucuparia, the European Mountain Ash, has red berries (Gaelic – *Caorann*). The American variety, *Sorbus americana*, has orange berries. The medicinal and edible qualities are the same.

The fruits of rowan have a very high quantity of vitamin C, which is why they were used in the Highlands for coughs, colds, bronchitis, and other lung afflictions. Highlanders simmered the berries with apples and honey to make a soothing syrup.

The berries (dried or fresh) can be simmered in water and then strained to make a vitamin C–rich gargle for sore throats and tonsillitis. For diarrhea, make rowan berry jelly. (Fresh berry juice is a mild laxative, but when cooked as jelly or jam the result is an astringent condiment that can relieve diarrhea.)

Highland ladies once wore necklaces of the berries as a form of magical protection. (Beith p. 237, Lust p. 339, Hopman, *Tree Medicine-Tree Magic* p. 81)

Rowan Berry Jelly

The nice thing is that the rowan berries and apples are ready at the same time of year.

2 pounds apples

2 pounds ripe rowan berries

3 tablespoons strained fresh lemon juice

Sugar or honey

(There is no need for pectin as rowan berries and apples already have it.)

Place the fruits into an enamel or glass cooking vessel and barely cover with cold water. Bring to a boil and simmer for about 40 minutes, stirring from time to time with a wooden spoon. (If froth develops at any time, an old trick is to add a tiny piece of butter to the pot. That will calm the froth.)

Add the lemon.

Make a jelly bag by hanging cheesecloth over a wooden hoop and pour the contents of the pot through the cloth into another container. Allow it to strain for six hours or longer. Do not squeeze the cloth or the jelly will be cloudy.

Measure the liquid that you have and add one cup of sugar (or slightly less honey) for every 1¼ cup of juice. To reduce cooking time, warm the sugar beforehand at 250 degree F. in an oven for 10 minutes.

Warm the liquid and add the warm sugar slowly, stirring with a wooden spoon until everything is dissolved. Boil until it reaches the jelling point, which is 250 degrees F. Test for the jelling point by putting a small amount in the refrigerator to see if it sets. Ladle into sterile jars and boil the jars briefly, loosely capped, to set the seal.

Heather

Heather (*Calluna vulgaris*, *Erica cinerea*, *Erica tetralix*) (Gaelic – *Fraoch*) tea can be applied to the head with a cloth for headache or for insomnia. Heather tea is soothing to the nerves, and the flowering tops can be used either fresh or dried. In old Scotland, pillows and mattresses were stuffed with heather to ensure restful sleep. The Picts (the indigenous pre-Celtic tribes of Scotland) added heather flowers to ale, which they made without the use of malt, hops, or any other sweetener.

A tea of the flowering tops will help coughs, calm the nerves, and benefit gout, rheumatic pains, and indigestion. The flowers are added to salves for arthritis and rheumatism. Heather strengthens the heart, is slightly diuretic, and slightly raises blood pressure (avoid heather if high blood pressure is a problem).

Heather tea helps to increase breast milk production. It can be helpful in cystitis as it is antimicrobial. A hot poultice of the flowers can be applied to chilblains. (Beith p. 222, Lust, p. 216, Livingstone p. 129)

Heather Tea

Steep 1 teaspoon of the flowering shoots in one half cup freshly boiled water for 10 minutes or simmer 4 teaspoons of the shoots in 1 cup of water for about 5 minutes. Take ¼ cup twice a day. Make a slightly stronger tea for external use as a headache compress.

Heather Ale

1	gallon heather (flowering tops)
2	pounds malt extract
1½	pounds sugar
3	gallons water
1	ounce yeast

Gather the heather tops when they are just coming into bloom. Boil the tops in 1 gallon of water for about an hour. Strain through a jelly bag (see rowan berry jelly instructions) onto the malt extract and sugar. Stir until dissolved. Add the rest of the water and, when lukewarm, the yeast.

(Recipe from: http://druidry.org/obod/trees/Heather.htm)

Atholl Brose

Brose (rhymes with rose) is a porridge-type dish of oatmeal or peasemeal prepared with boiling hot water, a pinch of salt and a bit of butter. Atholl Brose is something quite different—a drink with a puddinglike consistency to which heavy cream is sometimes added. This recipe was first recorded in 1475.

> 3   rounded tablespoons medium oatmeal
>
> 2   cups cold water
>
> 2   tablespoons heather honey
>
> 1   quart Scotch whisky (maximum)

Place the oats in a basin and mix with cold water until a thick paste consistency is achieved. Allow to sit for 30 minutes.

Force the oats through a fine strainer, pressing with a wooden spoon to extract the last bit of liquid.

Discard the solid oatmeal and save the creamy oatmeal liquid for the brose.

Mix 4 tablespoons of heather honey and 4 sherry glassfuls of the liquid oatmeal and stir with a silver spoon. Add heavy cream if desired. Pour the resulting liquid into a quart bottle and fill with malt whisky. Shake well and serve.

(from: http://www.rampantscotland.com/recipes/blrecipe _brose.htm)

Thistles

If one plant symbolizes all that is Scotland, this is it. Tough, persistent, gritty, and beautiful, the hardy thistle (*Onopordon acanthium, Cardus heterophyllus, Sonchus oleraceus*) (Gaelic – *gíogan, cluaran, cluas an fleidh*) thrives where other plants can only wither.

The root of Scotch thistle (*Onopordon acanthium*) is astringent and is used to purge mucus. Simmer 1 ounce of the root in 1½ pints of water until 1 pint remains. The fresh juice, which can be applied to cancerous tumors and ulcers, is also helpful for nervous complaints.

The melancholy thistle (*Cardus heterophyllus*) (Gaelic – *cluas an fleidh*) can be simmered in wine to dispel depression. (Beith, p. 246, Grieve, p. 798)

Sonchus oleraceus, the sow thistle, is a liver cleanser and emmenagogue. Steep the leaves and roots (not the stem) as a tea for fevers and to treat diarrhea. The leaves are used to poultice inflammations and swellings. Apply the sap to warts. (http://www.pfaf.org/database/plants.php?Sonchus+oleraceus)

Cooked Scotch Thistle

The flower buds can be eaten like artichokes and the stems are cooked like asparagus or rhubarb (peel before cooking). The young leaves can be picked before the flowers appear and cooked (remove the prickles before cooking). The petals can be mixed with saffron as a yellow food coloring and flavoring.

(From: www.pfaf.org/database/plants.php?Onopordum+acanthium)

Cooked Sow Thistle

The young leaves are tasty either raw or cooked. Add them to salads or use like spinach. Remove the prickles before cooking or eating. The stems can be cooked like asparagus or rhubarb (remove the outer skin first). According to reports, this thistle is the tastiest.

(From: www.pfaf.org/database/plants.php?Sonchus+oleraceus)

Sources Cited

Beith, Mary. *Healing Threads*. Edinburg: Polygon, 1995.

Grieve, M. *A Modern Herbal*, Vol. I, II. Dover Publications: New York, 1971.

Hopman, Ellen Evert, *A Druid's Herbal – For the Sacred Earth Year*, Rochester, VT: Destiny Books, 1995.

Hopman, Ellen Evert. *Tree Medicine-Tree Magic*. Custer, WA: Phoenix Publishing Inc., 1991.

Livingstone, Sheila. *Scottish Customs*. New York: Barnes and Noble Books, 1997.

Lust, John. *The Herb Book*. New York: Bantam Books, 1974.

Smith-Twiddy, Helen. *Celtic Cookbook*. Talybont, Ceredigion, Wales: Y Lolfa Cyf, 2002.

Web Sites Consulted

www.pfaf.org/database/plants.php?Onopordum+acanthium

www.pfaf.org/database/plants.php?Sonchus+oleraceus

www.rampantscotland.com/recipes/blrecipe_brose.htm

A Plate of Herbal Passion

⊰ by Nancy V. Bennett ⊱

For many generations, herbs have been a part of our lives, our plates, and our mythology, so it is no surprise that they have become part of our romantic rituals. Here are a few passionate offerings from the past to enhance and enchant you.

Anise at Your Wedding

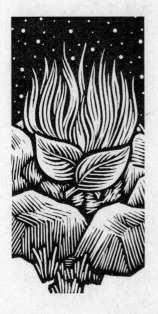

An herb as well as a spice, anise seeds were popular with ancient Romans and were used to make a spiced cake to be served at the end of a wedding feast. Anise is also effective protection against the evil eye, in case the in-laws didn't like you!

An all-purpose plant, the Romans also found anise to be a good aid to digestion with a wonderful licorice taste. If you wish to feel youthful and vibrant again, hang a sprig of anise on your bedpost. Sweet romantic dreams will also come if you place it under your pillow.

Basil

Herb of Kings and Teller of Fortunes

The Greeks had a passion for it, so much so that they named it from their root word *Basilikon*, meaning "royal" or "kingly." According to custom, the king himself would harvest the first basil with a golden sickle. Though both the Greeks and the Egyptians used the plant in their death rituals, for the Romans it was a symbol for love.

For Romanians, basil is also linked to the heart. In this country, when a man accepts a sprig of basil from a woman, they are engaged. In Italy, women with romance on their mind will place a pot of basil on their doorstep or patio to give a "come hither" sign to their beloved.

Want to test if your relationship is on track? Place two basil leaves onto a bed of coals. If they lie side by side and smolder together, then your future is secure. If they fly apart and burn separately, it may be time to look for another lover.

But do not fret. If you want to make sure you never lose that loving feeling, a healthy way to incorporate basil into your diet is to make your own fresh pesto.

Passion Pesto

2   cups fresh basil (packed)

4   tablespoons pine nuts, walnuts or almonds
    (traditionally pine nuts are used, but other
    nuts make nice variations)

½ – ⅔   cup olive oil (good olive oil recommended
    —it makes all the difference)

¼ – ⅓   cup grated Parmesan cheese

3   cloves of garlic

In a food processor, start with about ⅓ cup leaves and pulse until finely chopped. Add about ⅓ of the nuts, cheese, and garlic and pulse again. Drizzle in olive oil. Continue adding ingredients in that order (basil, nuts, cheese, and oil) until pesto is a smooth green paste.

Pesto can be used on everything from bread to chicken to pasta, or even stirred into soups. You can store the pesto in a well-sealed container in the fridge for about a week or for three months or so in the freezer.

Myrtle Makes Magic

Myrtle, though not as common in the household as bay leaves, is still used today in baking, marinating, and stews. It was once the herb made for lovers, especially during Venus' festival in Rome called the Venus Verticordia, when maidens would bathe in scented water and wear myrtle leaves in their hair.

As a symbol of love and fertility, bridesmaids in Wales were favored by a sprig of it from the bride to be. Before talcum powder became known, myrtle was used in a dried and powdered form on babies' bottoms.

Minerva changed one of her favorite followers into a myrtle bush to avoid a god's advances and preserve her virginity, and Venus used a similar bush to hide from roving Satyrs. It was also associated with death, and once was used to entice the goddess Persephone to release Bacchus' mother from the underworld.

Marjoram Most Misunderstood

Throughout history, marjoram and oregano have been mistaken for each other, but this herb deserves to stand on its own. In olden days, its uses included room fresheners, soaps, and sachets.

Attributed to Venus, who first grew it on Mount Ida, marjoram is the herb for a happy marriage and happy afterlife. In ancient times, you would find it in bridal wreaths as well as planted in graveyards. Crush a marjoram leaf and place its oil upon your forehead before going to bed and you will dream of a future lover.

Mint Sweet Minthe

It was a fateful day for the nymph named Minthe when the goddess Persephone caught her in the arms of Hades. Hades was already married to Persephone! The scorned and angry goddess Persephone trod Minthe into the ground. Hades had remorse over the sweet young thing's demise and changed her forever more into a mint plant.

In ancient times, followers of Bacchus would wear the mint plant in their hair to avoid getting too tipsy too fast. The sweet smell was useful for attracting a possible mate, and young maidens in attendance wove it into their hair at weddings. Mint was said to turn young men's thoughts to love, so much so that Alexander the Great was advised by Hippocrates not to let his soldiers drink mint tea before a battle.

Fenugreek, Sage, and Parsley

A passionate look at herbs would not be complete without adding a brief look at these three.

Fenugreek seeds were once used in harems to improve the buxomness and the overall appearance of the sultan's women. Sage tea was given to the returning soldiers in Greece by their wives, who were hoping to become pregnant. And finally, it was believed that Witches could not fly without using parsley rubbed on their brooms.

I hope you will find your passion for herbs, and enjoy all the bounty. So without further ado—one last recipe for you that I share with only special partners. May it fly a little romance into your evening.

1⅓ cup frozen spinach, chopped and thawed

1 cup ricotta cheese

¼ cup fresh parsley

1 tablespoon fresh chives, cut fine

1 large egg

1 teaspoon salt

1 package puff pastry, thawed

For the Filling:

Squeeze the excess liquid from the spinach and thoroughly mix in the ricotta cheese, parsley, chives, egg, and salt.

Preheat oven to 350 degrees F. Take 1 package puff pastry that has been thawed. Roll out half of the dough on a well-floured board and spread the filling on it evenly.

Then cover with second half of the dough, rolled to the same thickness.

Preparation:

There are two ways you can prepare this: The first is to simply score the top of the dough into squares or triangles, then cut through after baking. Or: using cookie cutters or a sharp knife, cut out different shapes. The best cutters are large ones with just a frame, as you will have to go through three layers. Always flour your cutter generously in between each use.

Bake until golden brown, 30 minutes if using the first full-sheet method and about 20 to 25 minutes for cut ones. I recommend using parchment paper on your cookie sheets. If not, keep a close eye on them so the bottoms do not burn.

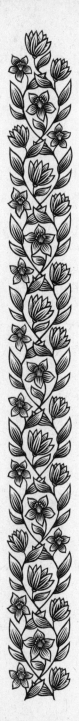

The
Quarters and
Signs of the
Moon and
Moon
Tables

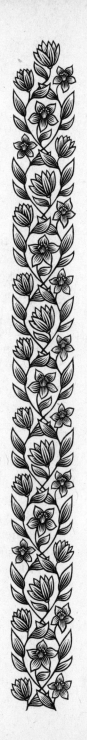

The Quarters and Signs
of the Moon

Everyone has seen the Moon wax and wane through a period of approximately twenty-nine-and-a-half days. This circuit from New Moon to Full Moon and back again is called the lunation cycle. The cycle is divided into parts called quarters or phases. There are several methods by which this can be done, and the system used in the *Herbal Almanac* may not correspond to those used in other almanacs.

The Quarters
First Quarter

The first quarter begins at the New Moon, when the Sun and Moon are in the same place, or conjunct. (This means that the Sun and Moon are in the same degree of the same sign.) The Moon is not visible at first, since it rises at the same time as the Sun. The New Moon is the time of new beginnings, beginnings of projects that favor growth, externalization of activities, and the growth of ideas. The first quarter is the time of germination, emergence, beginnings, and outwardly directed activity.

Second Quarter

The second quarter begins halfway between the New Moon and the Full Moon, when the Sun and Moon are at right angles, or a ninety-degree square to each other. This half Moon rises around noon and sets around midnight, so it can be seen in the western sky during the first half of the night. The second quarter is the time of growth and articulation of things that already exist.

Third Quarter

The third quarter begins at the Full Moon, when the Sun and Moon are opposite one another and the full light of the Sun can shine on the full sphere of the Moon. The round Moon can be seen rising in the east at sunset, and then rising a little later each evening. The Full Moon stands for illumination, fulfillment, culmination, completion, drawing inward, unrest, emotional expressions, and hasty actions leading to failure. The third quarter is a time of maturity, fruition, and the assumption of the full form of expression.

Fourth Quarter

The fourth quarter begins about halfway between the Full Moon and New Moon, when the Sun and Moon are again at ninety degrees, or square. This decreasing Moon rises at midnight and can be seen in the east during the last half of the night, reaching the overhead position just about as the Sun rises. The fourth quarter is a time of disintegration and drawing back for reorganization and reflection.

The Signs

Moon in Aries

Moon in Aries is good for starting things, but lacking in staying power. Things occur rapidly, but also quickly pass.

Moon in Taurus

With Moon in Taurus, things begun during this sign last the longest and tend to increase in value. Things begun now become habitual and hard to alter.

Moon in Gemini

Moon in Gemini is an inconsistent position for the Moon, characterized by a lot of talk. Things begun now are easily changed by outside influences.

Moon in Cancer

Moon in Cancer stimulates emotional rapport between people. It pinpoints need and supports growth and nurturance.

Moon in Leo

Moon in Leo accents showmanship, being seen, drama, recreation, and happy pursuits. It may be concerned with praise and subject to flattery.

Moon in Virgo

Moon in Virgo favors accomplishment of details and commands from higher up, while discouraging independent thinking.

Moon in Libra

Moon in Libra increases self-awareness. This moon favors self-examination and interaction with others, but discourages spontaneous initiative.

Moon in Scorpio

Moon in Scorpio increases awareness of psychic power. It precipitates psychic crises and ends connections thoroughly.

Moon in Sagittarius

Moon in Sagittarius encourages expansionary flights of imagination and confidence in the flow of life.

Moon in Capricorn

Moon in Capricorn increases awareness of the need for structure, discipline, and organization. Institutional activities are favored.

Moon in Aquarius

Moon in Aquarius favors activities that are unique and individualistic, concern for humanitarian needs and society as a whole, and improvements that can be made.

Moon in Pisces

During Moon in Pisces, energy withdraws from the surface of life and hibernates within, secretly reorganizing and realigning.

January Moon Table

Date	Sign	Element	Nature	Phase
1 Thu	Pisces	Water	Fruitful	1st
2 Fri	Pisces	Water	Fruitful	1st
3 Sat 4:50 am	Aries	Fire	Barren	1st
4 Sun	Aries	Fire	Barren	2nd 6:56 am
5 Mon 10:46 am	Taurus	Earth	Semi-fruitful	2nd
6 Tue	Taurus	Earth	Semi-fruitful	2nd
7 Wed 1:11 pm	Gemini	Air	Barren	2nd
8 Thu	Gemini	Air	Barren	2nd
9 Fri 1:14 pm	Cancer	Water	Fruitful	2nd
10 Sat	Cancer	Water	Fruitful	3rd 10:27 pm
11 Sun 12:41 pm	Leo	Fire	Barren	3rd
12 Mon	Leo	Fire	Barren	3rd
13 Tue 1:33 pm	Virgo	Earth	Barren	3rd
14 Wed	Virgo	Earth	Barren	3rd
15 Thu 5:30 pm	Libra	Air	Semi-fruitful	3rd
16 Fri	Libra	Air	Semi-fruitful	3rd
17 Sat	Libra	Air	Semi-fruitful	4th 9:46 pm
18 Sun 1:20 am	Scorpio	Water	Fruitful	4th
19 Mon	Scorpio	Water	Fruitful	4th
20 Tue 12:30 pm	Sagittarius	Fire	Barren	4th
21 Wed	Sagittarius	Fire	Barren	4th
22 Thu	Sagittarius	Fire	Barren	4th
23 Fri 1:18 am	Capricorn	Earth	Semi-fruitful	4th
24 Sat	Capricorn	Earth	Semi-fruitful	4th
25 Sun 1:56 pm	Aquarius	Air	Barren	4th
26 Mon	Aquarius	Air	Barren	1st 2:55 am
27 Tue	Aquarius	Air	Barren	1st
28 Wed 1:12 am	Pisces	Water	Fruitful	1st
29 Thu	Pisces	Water	Fruitful	1st
30 Fri 10:25 am	Aries	Fire	Barren	1st
31 Sat	Aries	Fire	Barren	1st

February Moon Table

Date	Sign	Element	Nature	Phase
1 Sun 5:08 pm	Taurus	Earth	Semi-fruitful	1st
2 Mon	Taurus	Earth	Semi-fruitful	2nd 6:13 pm
3 Tue 9:14 pm	Gemini	Air	Barren	2nd
4 Wed	Gemini	Air	Barren	2nd
5 Thu 11:05 pm	Cancer	Water	Fruitful	2nd
6 Fri	Cancer	Water	Fruitful	2nd
7 Sat 11:43 pm	Leo	Fire	Barren	2nd
8 Sun	Leo	Fire	Barren	2nd
9 Mon	Leo	Fire	Barren	3rd 9:49 am
10 Tue 12:38 am	Virgo	Earth	Barren	3rd
11 Wed	Virgo	Earth	Barren	3rd
12 Thu 3:33 am	Libra	Air	Semi-fruitful	3rd
13 Fri	Libra	Air	Semi-fruitful	3rd
14 Sat 9:50 am	Scorpio	Water	Fruitful	3rd
15 Sun	Scorpio	Water	Fruitful	3rd
16 Mon 7:53 pm	Sagittarius	Fire	Barren	4th 4:37 pm
17 Tue	Sagittarius	Fire	Barren	4th
18 Wed	Sagittarius	Fire	Barren	4th
19 Thu 8:25 am	Capricorn	Earth	Semi-fruitful	4th
20 Fri	Capricorn	Earth	Semi-fruitful	4th
21 Sat 9:06 pm	Aquarius	Air	Barren	4th
22 Sun	Aquarius	Air	Barren	4th
23 Mon	Aquarius	Air	Barren	4th
24 Tue 7:59 am	Pisces	Water	Fruitful	1st 8:35 pm
25 Wed	Pisces	Water	Fruitful	1st
26 Thu 4:24 pm	Aries	Fire	Barren	1st
27 Fri	Aries	Fire	Barren	1st
28 Sat 10:33 pm	Taurus	Earth	Semi-fruitful	1st

March Moon Table

Date	Sign	Element	Nature	Phase
1 Sun	Taurus	Earth	Semi-fruitful	1st
2 Mon	Taurus	Earth	Semi-fruitful	1st
3 Tue 2:59 am	Gemini	Air	Barren	1st
4 Wed	Gemini	Air	Barren	2nd 2:46 am
5 Thu 6:07 am	Cancer	Water	Fruitful	2nd
6 Fri	Cancer	Water	Fruitful	2nd
7 Sat 8:24 am	Leo	Fire	Barren	2nd
8 Sun	Leo	Fire	Barren	2nd
9 Mon 11:34 am	Virgo	Earth	Barren	2nd
10 Tue	Virgo	Earth	Barren	3rd 10:38 pm
11 Wed 2:46 pm	Libra	Air	Semi-fruitful	3rd
12 Thu	Libra	Air	Semi-fruitful	3rd
13 Fri 8:22 pm	Scorpio	Water	Fruitful	3rd
14 Sat	Scorpio	Water	Fruitful	3rd
15 Sun	Scorpio	Water	Fruitful	3rd
16 Mon 5:21 am	Sagittarius	Fire	Barren	3rd
17 Tue	Sagittarius	Fire	Barren	3rd
18 Wed 5:18 pm	Capricorn	Earth	Semi-fruitful	4th 1:47 pm
19 Thu	Capricorn	Earth	Semi-fruitful	4th
20 Fri	Capricorn	Earth	Semi-fruitful	4th
21 Sat 6:06 am	Aquarius	Air	Barren	4th
22 Sun	Aquarius	Air	Barren	4th
23 Mon 5:08 pm	Pisces	Water	Fruitful	4th
24 Tue	Pisces	Water	Fruitful	4th
25 Wed	Pisces	Water	Fruitful	4th
26 Thu 1:03 am	Aries	Fire	Barren	1st 12:06 am
27 Fri	Aries	Fire	Barren	1st
28 Sat 6:09 am	Taurus	Earth	Semi-fruitful	1st
29 Sun	Taurus	Earth	Semi-fruitful	1st
30 Mon 9:36 am	Gemini	Air	Barren	1st
31 Tue	Gemini	Air	Barren	1st

April Moon Table

Date	Sign	Element	Nature	Phase
1 Wed 12:30 pm	Cancer	Water	Fruitful	1st
2 Thu	Cancer	Water	Fruitful	2nd 10:34 am
3 Fri 3:32 pm	Leo	Fire	Barren	2nd
4 Sat	Leo	Fire	Barren	2nd
5 Sun 7:01 pm	Virgo	Earth	Barren	2nd
6 Mon	Virgo	Earth	Barren	2nd
7 Tue 11:22 pm	Libra	Air	Semi-fruitful	2nd
8 Wed	Libra	Air	Semi-fruitful	2nd
9 Thu	Libra	Air	Semi-fruitful	3rd 10:56 am
10 Fri 5:23 am	Scorpio	Water	Fruitful	3rd
11 Sat	Scorpio	Water	Fruitful	3rd
12 Sun 2:00 pm	Sagittarius	Fire	Barren	3rd
13 Mon	Sagittarius	Fire	Barren	3rd
14 Tue	Sagittarius	Fire	Barren	3rd
15 Wed 1:27 am	Capricorn	Earth	Semi-fruitful	3rd
16 Thu	Capricorn	Earth	Semi-fruitful	3rd
17 Fri 2:19 pm	Aquarius	Air	Barren	4th 9:36 am
18 Sat	Aquarius	Air	Barren	4th
19 Sun	Aquarius	Air	Barren	4th
20 Mon 1:55 am	Pisces	Water	Fruitful	4th
21 Tue	Pisces	Water	Fruitful	4th
22 Wed 10:09 am	Aries	Fire	Barren	4th
23 Thu	Aries	Fire	Barren	4th
24 Fri 2:46 pm	Taurus	Earth	Semi-fruitful	1st 11:22 pm
25 Sat	Taurus	Earth	Semi-fruitful	1st
26 Sun 5:02 pm	Gemini	Air	Barren	1st
27 Mon	Gemini	Air	Barren	1st
28 Tue 6:38 pm	Cancer	Water	Fruitful	1st
29 Wed	Cancer	Water	Fruitful	1st
30 Thu 8:56 pm	Leo	Fire	Barren	1st

May Moon Table

Date	Sign	Element	Nature	Phase
1 Fri	Leo	Fire	Barren	2nd 4:44 pm
2 Sat	Leo	Fire	Barren	2nd
3 Sun 12:37 am	Virgo	Earth	Barren	2nd
4 Mon	Virgo	Earth	Barren	2nd
5 Tue 5:51 am	Libra	Air	Semi-fruitful	2nd
6 Wed	Libra	Air	Semi-fruitful	2nd
7 Thu 12:48 pm	Scorpio	Water	Fruitful	2nd
8 Fri	Scorpio	Water	Fruitful	2nd
9 Sat 9:49 pm	Sagittarius	Fire	Barren	3rd 12:01 am
10 Sun	Sagittarius	Fire	Barren	3rd
11 Mon	Sagittarius	Fire	Barren	3rd
12 Tue 9:09 am	Capricorn	Earth	Semi-fruitful	3rd
13 Wed	Capricorn	Earth	Semi-fruitful	3rd
14 Thu 10:01 pm	Aquarius	Air	Barren	3rd
15 Fri	Aquarius	Air	Barren	3rd
16 Sat	Aquarius	Air	Barren	3rd
17 Sun 10:17 am	Pisces	Water	Fruitful	4th 3:26 am
18 Mon	Pisces	Water	Fruitful	4th
19 Tue 7:30 pm	Aries	Fire	Barren	4th
20 Wed	Aries	Fire	Barren	4th
21 Thu	Aries	Fire	Barren	4th
22 Fri 12:40 am	Taurus	Earth	Semi-fruitful	4th
23 Sat	Taurus	Earth	Semi-fruitful	4th
24 Sun 2:34 am	Gemini	Air	Barren	1st 8:11 am
25 Mon	Gemini	Air	Barren	1st
26 Tue 2:58 am	Cancer	Water	Fruitful	1st
27 Wed	Cancer	Water	Fruitful	1st
28 Thu 3:44 am	Leo	Fire	Barren	1st
29 Fri	Leo	Fire	Barren	1st
30 Sat 6:17 am	Virgo	Earth	Barren	2nd 11:22 pm
31 Sun	Virgo	Earth	Barren	2nd

June Moon Table

Date	Sign	Element	Nature	Phase
1 Mon 11:17 am	Libra	Air	Semi-fruitful	2nd
2 Tue	Libra	Air	Semi-fruitful	2nd
3 Wed 6:43 pm	Scorpio	Water	Fruitful	2nd
4 Thu	Scorpio	Water	Fruitful	2nd
5 Fri	Scorpio	Water	Fruitful	2nd
6 Sat 4:23 am	Sagittarius	Fire	Barren	2nd
7 Sun	Sagittarius	Fire	Barren	3rd 2:12 pm
8 Mon 3:59 pm	Capricorn	Earth	Semi-fruitful	3rd
9 Tue	Capricorn	Earth	Semi-fruitful	3rd
10 Wed	Capricorn	Earth	Semi-fruitful	3rd
11 Thu 4:52 am	Aquarius	Air	Barren	3rd
12 Fri	Aquarius	Air	Barren	3rd
13 Sat 5:32 pm	Pisces	Water	Fruitful	3rd
14 Sun	Pisces	Water	Fruitful	3rd
15 Mon	Pisces	Water	Fruitful	4th 6:14 pm
16 Tue 3:51 am	Aries	Fire	Barren	4th
17 Wed	Aries	Fire	Barren	4th
18 Thu 10:20 am	Taurus	Earth	Semi-fruitful	4th
19 Fri	Taurus	Earth	Semi-fruitful	4th
20 Sat 1:00 pm	Gemini	Air	Barren	4th
21 Sun	Gemini	Air	Barren	4th
22 Mon 1:12 pm	Cancer	Water	Fruitful	1st 3:35 pm
23 Tue	Cancer	Water	Fruitful	1st
24 Wed 12:50 pm	Leo	Fire	Barren	1st
25 Thu	Leo	Fire	Barren	1st
26 Fri 1:46 pm	Virgo	Earth	Barren	1st
27 Sat	Virgo	Earth	Barren	1st
28 Sun 5:24 pm	Libra	Air	Semi-fruitful	1st
29 Mon	Libra	Air	Semi-fruitful	2nd 7:28 am
30 Tue	Libra	Air	Semi-fruitful	2nd

July Moon Table

Date	Sign	Element	Nature	Phase
1 Wed 12:18 am	Scorpio	Water	Fruitful	2nd
2 Thu	Scorpio	Water	Fruitful	2nd
3 Fri 10:10 am	Sagittarius	Fire	Barren	2nd
4 Sat	Sagittarius	Fire	Barren	2nd
5 Sun 10:07 pm	Capricorn	Earth	Semi-fruitful	2nd
6 Mon	Capricorn	Earth	Semi-fruitful	2nd
7 Tue	Capricorn	Earth	Semi-fruitful	3rd 5:21 am
8 Wed 11:03 am	Aquarius	Air	Barren	3rd
9 Thu	Aquarius	Air	Barren	3rd
10 Fri 11:44 pm	Pisces	Water	Fruitful	3rd
11 Sat	Pisces	Water	Fruitful	3rd
12 Sun	Pisces	Water	Fruitful	3rd
13 Mon 10:40 am	Aries	Fire	Barren	3rd
14 Tue	Aries	Fire	Barren	3rd
15 Wed 6:30 pm	Taurus	Earth	Semi-fruitful	4th 5:53 am
16 Thu	Taurus	Earth	Semi-fruitful	4th
17 Fri 10:41 pm	Gemini	Air	Barren	4th
18 Sat	Gemini	Air	Barren	4th
19 Sun 11:51 pm	Cancer	Water	Fruitful	4th
20 Mon	Cancer	Water	Fruitful	4th
21 Tue 11:27 pm	Leo	Fire	Barren	1st 10:34 pm
22 Wed	Leo	Fire	Barren	1st
23 Thu 11:22 pm	Virgo	Earth	Barren	1st
24 Fri	Virgo	Earth	Barren	1st
25 Sat	Virgo	Earth	Barren	1st
26 Sun 1:25 am	Libra	Air	Semi-fruitful	1st
27 Mon	Libra	Air	Semi-fruitful	1st
28 Tue 6:56 am	Scorpio	Water	Fruitful	2nd 6:00 pm
29 Wed	Scorpio	Water	Fruitful	2nd
30 Thu 4:10 pm	Sagittarius	Fire	Barren	2nd
31 Fri	Sagittarius	Fire	Barren	2nd

August Moon Table

Date	Sign	Element	Nature	Phase
1 Sat	Sagittarius	Fire	Barren	2nd
2 Sun 4:08 am	Capricorn	Earth	Semi-fruitful	2nd
3 Mon	Capricorn	Earth	Semi-fruitful	2nd
4 Tue 5:08 pm	Aquarius	Air	Barren	2nd
5 Wed	Aquarius	Air	Barren	3rd 8:55 pm
6 Thu	Aquarius	Air	Barren	3rd
7 Fri 5:34 am	Pisces	Water	Fruitful	3rd
8 Sat	Pisces	Water	Fruitful	3rd
9 Sun 4:23 pm	Aries	Fire	Barren	3rd
10 Mon	Aries	Fire	Barren	3rd
11 Tue	Aries	Fire	Barren	3rd
12 Wed 12:49 am	Taurus	Earth	Semi-fruitful	3rd
13 Thu	Taurus	Earth	Semi-fruitful	4th 2:55 pm
14 Fri 6:25 am	Gemini	Air	Barren	4th
15 Sat	Gemini	Air	Barren	4th
16 Sun 9:13 am	Cancer	Water	Fruitful	4th
17 Mon	Cancer	Water	Fruitful	4th
18 Tue 9:56 am	Leo	Fire	Barren	4th
19 Wed	Leo	Fire	Barren	4th
20 Thu 10:00 am	Virgo	Earth	Barren	1st 6:01 am
21 Fri	Virgo	Earth	Barren	1st
22 Sat 11:12 am	Libra	Air	Semi-fruitful	1st
23 Sun	Libra	Air	Semi-fruitful	1st
24 Mon 3:16 pm	Scorpio	Water	Fruitful	1st
25 Tue	Scorpio	Water	Fruitful	1st
26 Wed 11:16 pm	Sagittarius	Fire	Barren	1st
27 Thu	Sagittarius	Fire	Barren	2nd 7:42 am
28 Fri	Sagittarius	Fire	Barren	2nd
29 Sat 10:44 am	Capricorn	Earth	Semi-fruitful	2nd
30 Sun	Capricorn	Earth	Semi-fruitful	2nd
31 Mon 11:43 pm	Aquarius	Air	Barren	2nd

September Moon Table

Date	Sign	Element	Nature	Phase
1 Tue	Aquarius	Air	Barren	2nd
2 Wed	Aquarius	Air	Barren	2nd
3 Thu 11:58 am	Pisces	Water	Fruitful	2nd
4 Fri	Pisces	Water	Fruitful	3rd 12:02 pm
5 Sat 10:14 pm	Aries	Fire	Barren	3rd
6 Sun	Aries	Fire	Barren	3rd
7 Mon	Aries	Fire	Barren	3rd
8 Tue 6:17 am	Taurus	Earth	Semi-fruitful	3rd
9 Wed	Taurus	Earth	Semi-fruitful	3rd
10 Thu 12:17 pm	Gemini	Air	Barren	3rd
11 Fri	Gemini	Air	Barren	4th 10:16 pm
12 Sat 4:19 pm	Cancer	Water	Fruitful	4th
13 Sun	Cancer	Water	Fruitful	4th
14 Mon 6:39 pm	Leo	Fire	Barren	4th
15 Tue	Leo	Fire	Barren	4th
16 Wed 7:56 pm	Virgo	Earth	Barren	4th
17 Thu	Virgo	Earth	Barren	4th
18 Fri 9:26 pm	Libra	Air	Semi-fruitful	1st 2:44 pm
19 Sat	Libra	Air	Semi-fruitful	1st
20 Sun	Libra	Air	Semi-fruitful	1st
21 Mon 12:52 am	Scorpio	Water	Fruitful	1st
22 Tue	Scorpio	Water	Fruitful	1st
23 Wed 7:43 am	Sagittarius	Fire	Barren	1st
24 Thu	Sagittarius	Fire	Barren	1st
25 Fri 6:19 pm	Capricorn	Earth	Semi-fruitful	1st
26 Sat	Capricorn	Earth	Semi-fruitful	2nd 12:50 am
27 Sun	Capricorn	Earth	Semi-fruitful	2nd
28 Mon 7:06 am	Aquarius	Air	Barren	2nd
29 Tue	Aquarius	Air	Barren	2nd
30 Wed 7:26 pm	Pisces	Water	Fruitful	2nd

October Moon Table

Date	Sign	Element	Nature	Phase
1 Thu	Pisces	Water	Fruitful	2nd
2 Fri	Pisces	Water	Fruitful	2nd
3 Sat 5:20 am	Aries	Fire	Barren	2nd
4 Sun	Aries	Fire	Barren	3rd 2:10 am
5 Mon 12:33 pm	Taurus	Earth	Semi-fruitful	3rd
6 Tue	Taurus	Earth	Semi-fruitful	3rd
7 Wed 5:46 pm	Gemini	Air	Barren	3rd
8 Thu	Gemini	Air	Barren	3rd
9 Fri 9:48 pm	Cancer	Water	Fruitful	3rd
10 Sat	Cancer	Water	Fruitful	3rd
11 Sun	Cancer	Water	Fruitful	4th 4:56 am
12 Mon 1:02 am	Leo	Fire	Barren	4th
13 Tue	Leo	Fire	Barren	4th
14 Wed 3:45 am	Virgo	Earth	Barren	4th
15 Thu	Virgo	Earth	Barren	4th
16 Fri 6:29 am	Libra	Air	Semi-fruitful	4th
17 Sat	Libra	Air	Semi-fruitful	4th
18 Sun 10:22 am	Scorpio	Water	Fruitful	1st 1:33 am
19 Mon	Scorpio	Water	Fruitful	1st
20 Tue 4:49 pm	Sagittarius	Fire	Barren	1st
21 Wed	Sagittarius	Fire	Barren	1st
22 Thu	Sagittarius	Fire	Barren	1st
23 Fri 2:39 am	Capricorn	Earth	Semi-fruitful	1st
24 Sat	Capricorn	Earth	Semi-fruitful	1st
25 Sun 3:08 pm	Aquarius	Air	Barren	2nd 8:42 pm
26 Mon	Aquarius	Air	Barren	2nd
27 Tue	Aquarius	Air	Barren	2nd
28 Wed 3:45 am	Pisces	Water	Fruitful	2nd
29 Thu	Pisces	Water	Fruitful	2nd
30 Fri 1:56 pm	Aries	Fire	Barren	2nd
31 Sat	Aries	Fire	Barren	2nd

November Moon Table

Date	Sign	Element	Nature	Phase
1 Sun 7:44 pm	Taurus	Earth	Semi-fruitful	2nd
2 Mon	Taurus	Earth	Semi-fruitful	3rd 2:14 pm
3 Tue 11:53 pm	Gemini	Air	Barren	3rd
4 Wed	Gemini	Air	Barren	3rd
5 Thu	Gemini	Air	Barren	3rd
6 Fri 2:42 am	Cancer	Water	Fruitful	3rd
7 Sat	Cancer	Water	Fruitful	3rd
8 Sun 5:23 am	Leo	Fire	Barren	3rd
9 Mon	Leo	Fire	Barren	4th 10:56 am
10 Tue 8:30 am	Virgo	Earth	Barren	4th
11 Wed	Virgo	Earth	Barren	4th
12 Thu 12:22 pm	Libra	Air	Semi-fruitful	4th
13 Fri	Libra	Air	Semi-fruitful	4th
14 Sat 5:24 pm	Scorpio	Water	Fruitful	4th
15 Sun	Scorpio	Water	Fruitful	4th
16 Mon	Scorpio	Water	Fruitful	1st 2:14 pm
17 Tue 12:22 am	Sagittarius	Fire	Barren	1st
18 Wed	Sagittarius	Fire	Barren	1st
19 Thu 10:00 am	Capricorn	Earth	Semi-fruitful	1st
20 Fri	Capricorn	Earth	Semi-fruitful	1st
21 Sat 10:11 pm	Aquarius	Air	Barren	1st
22 Sun	Aquarius	Air	Barren	1st
23 Mon	Aquarius	Air	Barren	1st
24 Tue 11:07 am	Pisces	Water	Fruitful	2nd 4:39 pm
25 Wed	Pisces	Water	Fruitful	2nd
26 Thu 10:10 pm	Aries	Fire	Barren	2nd
27 Fri	Aries	Fire	Barren	2nd
28 Sat	Aries	Fire	Barren	2nd
29 Sun 5:34 am	Taurus	Earth	Semi-fruitful	2nd
30 Mon	Taurus	Earth	Semi-fruitful	2nd

December Moon Table

Date	Sign	Element	Nature	Phase
1 Tue 9:23 am	Gemini	Air	Barren	2nd
2 Wed	Gemini	Air	Barren	3rd 2:30 am
3 Thu 11:00 am	Cancer	Water	Fruitful	3rd
4 Fri	Cancer	Water	Fruitful	3rd
5 Sat 12:07 pm	Leo	Fire	Barren	3rd
6 Sun	Leo	Fire	Barren	3rd
7 Mon 2:05 pm	Virgo	Earth	Barren	3rd
8 Tue	Virgo	Earth	Barren	4th 7:13 pm
9 Wed 5:47 pm	Libra	Air	Semi-fruitful	4th
10 Thu	Libra	Air	Semi-fruitful	4th
11 Fri 11:31 pm	Scorpio	Water	Fruitful	4th
12 Sat	Scorpio	Water	Fruitful	4th
13 Sun	Scorpio	Water	Fruitful	4th
14 Mon 7:25 am	Sagittarius	Fire	Barren	4th
15 Tue	Sagittarius	Fire	Barren	4th
16 Wed 5:32 pm	Capricorn	Earth	Semi-fruitful	1st 7:02 am
17 Thu	Capricorn	Earth	Semi-fruitful	1st
18 Fri	Capricorn	Earth	Semi-fruitful	1st
19 Sat 5:38 am	Aquarius	Air	Barren	1st
20 Sun	Aquarius	Air	Barren	1st
21 Mon 6:42 pm	Pisces	Water	Fruitful	1st
22 Tue	Pisces	Water	Fruitful	1st
23 Wed	Pisces	Water	Fruitful	1st
24 Thu 6:39 am	Aries	Fire	Barren	2nd 12:36 pm
25 Fri	Aries	Fire	Barren	2nd
26 Sat 3:26 pm	Taurus	Earth	Semi-fruitful	2nd
27 Sun	Taurus	Earth	Semi-fruitful	2nd
28 Mon 8:13 pm	Gemini	Air	Barren	2nd
29 Tue	Gemini	Air	Barren	2nd
30 Wed 9:45 pm	Cancer	Water	Fruitful	2nd
31 Thu	Cancer	Water	Fruitful	3rd 2:13 pm

About the Authors

ELIZABETH BARRETTE serves as the managing editor of *PanGaia*. The central Illinois resident has been involved with the Pagan community for more than seventeen years. Her other writing fields include speculative fiction and gender studies. Visit her Web site at www.worthlink.net/~ysabet/sitemap.html

CHANDRA MOIRA BEAL is a freelance writer currently living in England. She has authored three books and published hundreds of articles, all inspired by her day-to-day life and adventures. She has been writing for Llewellyn since 1998. Chandra is also a massage therapist. To learn more, visit www.beal-net.com/laluna

NANCY V. BENNETT has been published in Llewellyn's annuals, *We'moon*, *Circle Network*, and many mainstream publications. Her pet projects include reading and writing about history and creating ethnic dinners to test on her family.

KRYSTAL BOWDEN, who has been studying the magical and mundane properties of herbs and essential oils for over ten years, has written articles on herbalism, aromatherapy, and natural living for the past six years. She has been the coordinator of the Circle of Gaia Dreaming for four years and also presents workshops relating to Paganism. She lives in Ohio with her partner, young son, five cats, and a dog.

CALANTIRNIEL has worked with herbs and natural healing since the early 1990s and became a certified Master Herbalist in 2007. She lives in Western Montana with her husband and daughter while her son is off to college. She also manages to have an organic garden and crochets professionally. Find out more at www.myspace.com/aartiana

KAAREN CHRIST is a consultant providing research and writing services to social service organizations. She also writes children's stories and crafts poetry. She lives in Prince Edward County, Ontario, with two beautiful children (Indigo and Challian), a Super-Dog called Lukki, and a magical boy-rabbit.

DALLAS JENNIFER COBB lives in an enchanted waterfront village where she focuses on what she loves: family, gardens, fitness, and fabulous food. Her essays are in Llewellyn's almanacs and recent Seal Press anthologies *Three Ring Circus* and *Far From Home*. Her video documentary, *Disparate Places*, appeared on TV Ontario's Planet Parent. Contact her at Jennifer.Cobb@Sympatico.ca

SALLY CRAGIN writes the astrological forecast, "Moon Signs," for the *Boston Phoenix*, which is syndicated throughout New England. She can also be heard on several radio stations as "Symboline Dai." A regular arts reviewer and feature writer for the *Boston Globe*, she also edits *Button, New England's Tiniest Magazine of Poetry, Fiction, and Gracious Living*. For more, including your personal forecast that clients have called "scary-accurate," see http://moonsigns.net

CLEA DANAAN is the author of *Sacred Land: Intuitive Gardening for Personal, Political & Environmental Change* (Llewellyn, 2007). She lives in Colorado with her daughter and husband, two spoiled cats, and an herb garden.

SORITA D'ESTE is an author and esoteric researcher who lives and works in Wales (UK) with her author partner David Rankine. Her published works include *The Guises of Morrigan, Hekate—Keys to the Crossroads*, and *Avalonia's Book of Chakras*. She facilitates workshops and gives regular lectures on subjects ranging from astral projection to herbalism, magic, and mythology. For more information, visit www.avalonia.co.uk

ALICE DEVILLE is an internationally known astrologer, writer, and metaphysical consultant. She has been both a reiki and seichim master since 1996. In her northern Virginia practice, Alice specializes in relationships, health, healing, real estate, government affairs, career and change management, and spiritual development. Contact Alice at DeVilleAA@aol.com

EMBER is a freelance writer, poet, and regular contributor to Llewellyn annuals. She enjoys hiking, photography, gardening, and anything that keeps her in touch with Mother Nature. She lives in Missouri with her husband of thirteen years and two feline companions.

MAGENTA GRIFFITH, a Witch for nearly thirty years, was in 1980 a founding member of the coven Prodea. She has been a member of the Covenant of the Goddess, CUUPs, Church of All Worlds, and several other Pagan organizations. She presents workshops and classes at festivals and gatherings around the Midwest.

CHERYL HOARD has studied herbalism and aromatherapy since 1976, been president of the National Association for Holistic Aromatherapy (NAHA) twice, and served as a complementary health lecturer for several colleges. Since 1991 she has been owner of Cheryl's Herbs, an international wholesale/retail/mail order supplier of over 5,000 highest quality herbal and aromatherapy products—with the goal of making it easier for you to have a more natural and healthy lifestyle.

ELLEN EVERT HOPMAN, herbalist, author, and Druid Priestess, is the author of *Priestess of the Forest: A Druid Novel* (Llewellyn, 2008). For more information, see her books, videos, and audio tapes at www.celticheritage.co.uk/EllenEvertHopman

JAMES KAMBOS is a writer and painter who has had a lifelong interest in folk magic. He has written numerous articles concerning the folk magic traditions of Greece, the Near East, and the Appalachian region of the United States. He writes and paints from his home in the beautiful Appalachian hills of southern Ohio.

KRISTIN MADDEN is a best-selling author of several books on parenting, shamanism, and paganism, including the Llewellyn books *The Book of Shamanic Healing* and *Dancing the Goddess Incarnate.* A Druid and tutor in the Order of Bards, Ovates, and

Druids, she is also Dean of the Ardantane School of Shamanic Studies. Kristin's work has appeared in print, on radio, and television in North America and Europe. She is also a homeschooling mom, wildlife rehabilitator, and environmental educator.

LISA MCSHERRY, a practicing Witch for more than twenty-five years, is the author of *Magickal Connections: Creating a Healthy and Lasting Spiritual Group* (New Page, 2007) and *The Virtual Pagan: Exploring Wicca and Paganism Through the Internet* (Weiser, 2002). The senior editor and owner of Facing North: A Community Resource (www.facingnorth.net) she is also a frequent contributor to Pagan publications. You can contact her at lisa@cybercoven.org

SUE J. MORRIS, founder and creator of Sue's Salves, combines her knowledge of organic gardening, natural healing, medical herbalism, nutrition, and astrology. Sue focuses on connecting the energies of the planets with the medicinal properties of plants. Sue also publishes a Planting by the Moon calendar, a day-to-day guide for all gardening activities based on the lunation cycle. Sue resides in central Pennsylvania, where she grows all of the plants for her line of products. Visit her Web site at www.suesalves.com

DANNY PHARR is an author and instructor. He is also the founder of the Wings of Fire Seminars, which provides individuals with a safe environment to discover joy, encourage personal achievement and growth, and engage in life-changing experiences. His first book, *The Moon and Everyday Living*, was published in 2000.

SUSANNA REPPERT operates The Rosemary House, an herb shop in Mechanicsburg, Pennsylvania, with her husband David. She learned the herb business from her mother, the store's founder, and has continued to learn more about the amazing and practical uses for plants. Susanna has recently completed an herbal medicine course at David Winston's Herbal Therapeutics School of Botanical Medicine.

SUZANNE RESS has been writing nonfiction and fiction for an eclectic array of publications for twenty-five years. She is an accomplished self-taught gardener and silversmith/mosaicist. She lives in the woods at the foot of the Alps in northern Italy with her husband, two teenage daughters, wolf dog, and two horses.

ANNE SALA is a freelance journalist based in Minnesota. She has been interested in herbs ever since she was a toddler, when her mother let her gather dill weed from the pot on the windowsill.

JANICE SHARKEY is an aromatherapist and keen astrological gardener. She loves scented plants and most of all, herbs. When she's not gardening, she's making stained glass panels or writing. One of her ambitions is to get her children David and Rose and her husband William to spend more time in the garden.

MICHELLE SKYE has been a practicing Witch for nine years. A founding member of the Sisterhood of the Crescent Moon, she is active in the southeastern Massachusetts Pagan community, presenting various workshops, classes, and apprenticeship programs. An ordained minister (Universal Life Church), she performs legal handfastings, weddings, and other spiritual rites of passage.

ZAEDA YIN is three-quarters Chinese, a tad Irish, and a lifelong solitary eclectic Pagan. She has lived, studied, and traveled extensively in India, Nepal, Japan, Hong Kong, Taiwan, Singapore, Malaysia, Thailand, and Borneo. Now based in Australia, her time is divided between writing and teaching the use of crystals, holy beads, and sacred objects from India and the Himalayas.

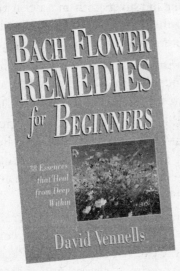

38 Essences that Heal from Deep Within

Bach Flower Remedies work on our subtle mental and emotional levels, where illness actually begins. They target the particular negative states of mind that give rise to the physical symptoms. You do not need a medical background to safely and effectively use these 38 different remedies for yourself, friends, family, and even pets.

**BACH FLOWER REMEDIES
FOR BEGINNERS**
312 pp. • 5³⁄₁₆ x 8
978-0-7387-0047-2 • U.S. $12.95 Can $19.95
To order call 1-877-NEW-WRLD
www.llewellyn.com

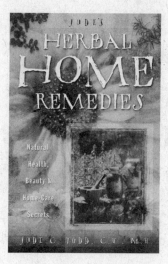

Natural Health, Beauty, and Home Care Secrets

Discover how cayenne pepper promotes hair growth, why cranberry juice is good for asthma attacks, how to make a potent juice to flush out fat, what herbs to use to rid your pet of fleas, and much more. This simple guide to self-care provides herbalists with advice for family, pets, garden, and household. Eight hundred remedies in all.

**JUDE'S HERBAL
HOME REMEDIES**
384 pp. • 6 x 9
978-0-8754-2869-7 • U.S. $16.95 Can $18.95
To order call 1-877-NEW-WRLD
www.llewellyn.com

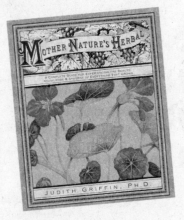

A Complete Guide to Everything that Grows

With ancient folklore, simple instructions for growing an herb garden, and recipes from around the world, *Mother Nature's Herbal* is hands down the most unique, thoughtful, and comprehensive guide to growing and preparing herbs. Graced with illustrations, this book presents centuries-old customs, gardening tips, and recipes for foods, teas, tonics, ointments, and medicines.

MOTHER NATURE'S HERBAL
432 pp. • 7½ x 9⅛
978-0-7387-1256-7 • U.S. $24.95 Can $28.95
To order call 1-877-NEW-WRLD
www.llewellyn.com